Spir

"*Spiritual Aging* places old age in the only perspective that gives it meaning and purpose, as one of our most prized privileges, a space and time to experience life from a brighter and higher perspective. Orsborn does not gloss over the difficulties and challenges of old age but incorporates them into her welcome vision, which helps us to embrace life, living, and ourselves. . . . This book is the honest, lived experience of one who walks her talk."

KAMLA K. KAPUR, AUTHOR OF
THE PRIVILEGE OF AGING

"Carol Orsborn harvests the deep wisdom of life's final act. Through extensive research, keen observation, archetypal symbolism and transpersonal experience, and her own exemplary personal growth, she shows us that we are the path we've been seeking. Intuitive, honest, and uncanny, this book gives you exactly what you need before you knew you needed it. Begin anywhere, stay for the rest of your life."

JOHN C. ROBINSON, AUTHOR OF
THE THREE SECRETS OF AGING

"A beautiful, beautiful book of weekly reflections. These delicious nuggets of deep wisdom, gentle respectfulness, and down-to-earth, heartfelt humanity call me to keep reading more. Highly recommended."

RICHARD MATZKIN, AUTHOR OF *LOVE AND TIME*

Spiritual Aging

WEEKLY REFLECTIONS FOR EMBRACING LIFE

Carol Orsborn, Ph.D.

Park Street Press
Rochester, Vermont

Park Street Press
One Park Street
Rochester, Vermont 05767
www.ParkStPress.com

Park Street Press is a division of Inner Traditions International

Select passages in this book have been adapted from Carol Orsborn's
previous books and blogs.

Cataloging-in-Publication Data for this title is available from the Library
of Congress

ISBN 978-1-64411-667-8 (print)
ISBN 978-1-64411-668-5 (ebook)

Printed and bound in the United States by Sheridan

10 9 8 7 6 5 4 3 2 1

Text design and layout by Kenleigh Manseau
This book was typeset in Garamond Premier Pro with Span and Myriad
pro used as display fonts

To send correspondence to the author of this book, mail a first-class
letter to the author c/o Inner Traditions • Bear & Company, One Park
Street, Rochester, VT 05767, and we will forward the communication,
or contact the author directly at **CarolOrsborn.com**.

Scan the QR code and save 25% at InnerTraditions.com.
Browse over 2,000 titles on spirituality, the occult, ancient
mysteries, new science, holistic health, and natural medicine.

To you, my beloved tribe of fierce old souls.
Thank you for keeping me company on this at
once most perilous and passionate stretch of our
journey through life.

Contents

THE READINGS
A PERENNIAL LOOP OF TWO-YEAR CYCLES

Foreword

Harry R. Moody, Ph.D.

Carol and I met fifteen years ago at the American Society of Aging, where we had each presented papers on our areas of expertise. I was the author of a textbook in gerontology, now in its tenth edition, and at the time Carol was applying her doctorate in life-stage theory, along with her multiple books on aging, to help such companies as AT&T and Ford target older market segments.

Now at ages seventy-nine and seventy-six, respectively, we not only study and teach about the demographic; we are part of it. That, and the fact that we have continued our lively conversations over the years about our shared interests, certainly qualifies us as old friends.

Carol uses this descriptor "old" throughout the weekly readings in this book. This is a gutsy move on her part, for in a culture that reveres youth, no one in the aging field ever grows "old," or if they do, they keep quiet about it. You'll never see elder gerontologists at conferences speaking from first-person experience. So instead we say "growing older," but not "old." As I said to someone recently, when asked about my retirement, I feel like a professor of Japanese who spent his whole career teaching the subject, and when he retired was able to visit Japan for the first time.

Carol's book is unapologetic in its appreciation of late life as an opportunity for conscious aging, a convergence of psychology and spirituality that turns upside down the mainstream paradigm privileging youth over old age. Viewed through the lens of spiritual aging, old age is perceived as holding the potential to be a culmination rather than a coda. As Carl Jung put it: "A human being would certainly not grow to be seventy or eighty years old if this longevity had no meaning for the species."

Spiritual aging argues that the primary task of development in the second half of life is to achieve some degree of detachment from all the busyness, frenzy, and overactivity that defines success in earlier life stages to make space for new life to emerge. In the words of Thomas Merton: "The greatest need of our time is to clean out the enormous mass of mental and emotional rubbish that clutters our minds."

It takes time, patience, and the willingness to be alone and vulnerable in order to refrain from turning our eyes away from what we fear about aging and be open to both the shadows and the wonders to be found on the far side of disillusionment. True creativity in later life demands not only letting go of what we've outgrown but the initiation of a journey into the wilderness to discover something in us that is wild and untamed. This is the process also described by Rabbi Zalman Schachter-Shalomi as "sage-ing," and by gerontologist

Lars Tornstam as "gerotranscendence."

Carving out time and space for deeper reflection is where Carol's newest book becomes an invaluable aid. Consisting of a perennial loop of weekly readings in a two-year cycle, the book is meant to be digested slowly and deeply. It invites readers to access a higher wisdom than is otherwise available to anticipate every conceivable mood, challenge, and topic they may encounter, "from transforming loneliness to solitude, loss of identity to freedom, anger to self-protection, envy to love," and more.

As Carol writes in her introduction, these readings "came to me from depths and sources beyond my ordinary consciousness in answer to my call for affirmation, insight, and guidance." Her deeper sources included a thousand dreams she experienced, recorded, and analyzed over a seven-year period.

In addition to our mutual interest in adult and spiritual development theory, an abiding interest in dreamwork is something we share, particularly in relation to aging. For fifteen years I have been researching the subject and have led numerous sessions on dreams at conferences in the aging field. The book I am writing on the subject shares research and examples of dreamwork as an entryway into the deeper levels of consciousness Carol's book brings to the surface to share with readers.

While you won't find the unprocessed symbols or narratives from her dreams in her readings (Carol stripped them out to more directly communicate the messages they carried), it is clear that her work is informed by such archetypal figures as what Jung called the Wise Old Man (*Senex,* in Latin) and Wise Old Woman. Think of Gandalf in *The Lord of the Rings,* or Obi-Wan Kenobi in *Star Wars.* As guide figures these wise old men and women may appear symbolically in dreams to serve as the source of visionary or prophetic truth during periods of confusion or uncertainty, especially at times when we need help in decision-making. Dreaming about these archetypes can express the dreamer's aspiration toward awareness of larger meaning in late life. Their appearance in dreams represents more than individual attitudes toward age. They also reflect ideals of wisdom and maturity, a totality and integral wholeness of being that we aspire to over the entire course of our lives.

The depth and creativity in Carol's readings stand on their own. Whether or not you are drawn to doing your own dreamwork, Carol's readings resonate with all of us who share her sincere willingness to respond to the deepest questions of life that emerge for us in old age.

Hold onto this book. Open it and read this week's entry or turn to any page at random. Then look in the mirror, both the physical mirror and the mirror of the mind. Ask yourself the questions: *Who are you? What do you already possess? What else is there to know?*

No matter your particular circumstances, spiritual aging holds the possibility of your becoming the person you were meant to be. This book is destined to become a generational classic, finding its home on bedside tables for years to come.

Harry (Rick) Moody, Ph.D., retired as vice president for academic affairs with AARP and is currently visiting faculty in the Creative Longevity and Wisdom Program at Fielding Graduate University and visiting professor at Tohoku University in Japan. He previously served as executive director of the Brookdale Center on Aging at Hunter College and chairman of the board of Elderhostel (now Road Scholar).

Moody is the author of *Ethics in an Aging Society*, the first book published on biomedical ethics and aging, and his forthcoming *Climate Change in an Aging Society* will be published by Routledge. He is coauthor of both *Aging: Concepts and Controversies*, a gerontology textbook now in its tenth edition, and *The Five Stages of the Soul*, which has been translated into seven languages. His *Human Values in Aging* newsletter has 5,000 subscribers monthly. In 2011 Moody received the Lifetime Achievement Award from the American Society on Aging. He lives in San Mateo, California.

Acknowledgments

To my children and grandchildren and our extended and growing family of beloved people and dogs—Grant, Ginny, Jody, Diego, Mason, Dylan, Winnie, Capi, and so many more—for sharing life and love with us and providing endless entertainment. And Dan, my *beshert*: fifty-six years! How wonderful it is to be growing old together.

Massive thanks to my agent and friend Linda Roghaar for introducing me to Inner Traditions years ago and to my brilliant editor Jamaica Burns Griffin and the inspired team at Inner Traditions, including Aaron Davis, Ashley Kolesnik, Abigail Lewis, Maria Loftus, Kenleigh Manseau, and Erica Robinson. Your passion for your work expresses itself in every detail. A special shout-out to Jon Graham, Jeanie Levitan, and Manzanita Carpenter Sanz for being among the first to take the plunge into the spiritual aging genre with Robert L. Weber's and my book, *The Spirituality of Age*, ten years ago; for staying faithful to the demographic against the tides of ageism in mainstream publishing; and for once again breaking new ground with *Spiritual Aging*'s unapologetic view of old age as culmination, which Rick Moody calls "a gutsy move."

Along these same lines, thanks, too, to Rosemary Cox at Sage-ing International, Dana Sue Walker of Spirit of Sophia, James Hollis, Rick Moody and the *Human Values in Aging Newsletter*, and Vanderbilt Divinity School for your continued and visionary support.

A grateful bow to Bob Weber and to the way-showers in my circle of friends, theologians, and guides, many of whom are quoted in this book. And especially to my soul sisters (and their significant others)—Marika Schoenberger, Deb Wick, Jill Speering, Judith Wolf-Mandell, Susan Edwards, Concon Medina, Alice Bryant, Liz Seibert, Fonda Lewis, Mary Beth Speer, Sue Stein, and Leean Nemeroff—for keeping me going through all the ups and downs of the fully lived life and for sharing your stories and dreams with me.

A heartfelt show of respect for my body, mind, and spirit support team: John Peach, Mark Thomasson, Lj Ratliff, Byron Stephens, Jed Maslow, Sandy Murphy, Kathleen Phillips and the leadership at Fifty Forward Madison Station, and Lois Wilson and my beloved friends at Serenity II.

And finally, to my mentor and friend, Connie Goldman, and to Mom and Dad—you would have liked this one.

My gratitude to you all is fierce, indeed.

Greetings, Old Friend

You and I have been working spiritually and psychologically for a long time to get to this place of arrival. We who have been transformed by the challenges of time have tasted the wholeness, freedom, and completion that is life's promise to us. We count ourselves fortunate to walk arm-in-arm with our cohort of lifelong seekers following the path of the mystics, elders, and old souls who have lit the way: Ram Dass, Rumi, Pema Chodron, and Carl Jung, to name a few. The growing cadre of way-showers grows deep and strong as we have learned from them so much about humility, acceptance, human nature, and what it means to fully embrace life.

In many ways the rewards wrested from growing older are greater than we'd ever expected. But even here, advancing toward the peak of adult and spiritual development, rising to meet life's many occasions is sometimes more than we can bear. Just when we begin to celebrate a degree of mastery, something unexpected raises the bar. We encounter old wounds we thought we'd made peace with long ago. The thing we were most afraid of knocks at the door. Or we simply forget for a time how small we are and how big the mystery. One of the ironies of age is that past levels of mastery will never prove sufficient because as we expand and deepen our consciousness, the questions become only larger.

This book of readings has come to you at this particular bend in the road to meet you wherever you are in your journey through life. Every week for the next two years and beyond you will be reminded how far you have come already, and that regardless of what life brings your way, you are never truly lost or alone.

The weekly readings comprise a perennial loop of two-year cycles meant to accompany you through the coming years. They are designed to be read one each week, your choice of day and time, and over every two years' span to cover every conceivable mood, challenge, and topic you may encounter. The readings are at once personal and archetypal, applicable to every one of us. They came to me from depths and sources beyond my ordinary consciousness in answer to my call for affirmation, insight, and guidance.

I literally lived, breathed, and dreamed these readings over the past seven years as I spent every morning recalling learnings gleaned from the most recent of more than a thousand dreams. This period included the marriage of my daughter and several years of solitude, first enforced by Covid, then by choice. Family and friends moved away for many good reasons. My husband and I understood, but still left us missing people we love, including our beloved grandchildren.

Along the way there was Dan's and my joyous fiftieth anniversary celebration and a new puppy, but there was also my own serious fall, surgery, and recovery. My fascination with my dream life sustained me through the highs and lows, and I came to view this period as the call to live even more deeply.

For the many of you who have put my books on bestseller lists in the aging category, you will have the opportunity to connect with this new material as well as revisit some favorite passages adapted to this new context from my previous work. All of the readings, referencing many of the thought leaders who have served as my influences, are informed by my years as a scholar in the fields of religion and adult and spiritual development, as well as my immersion in the works and practices of a wide range of mystic and spiritual traditions, past and present.

In keeping with the intuitive nature of inner work, while the readings subtly build upon one another, they are not linear. Rather, they circle back in sometimes expanding, sometimes contracting spirals until every facet of the major themes of spiritual aging has had the opportunity to be assimilated by the reader on multiple levels. A major influence on my life and this book is Carl Jung's assertion that the purpose of life is "increasing consciousness."

Jung also asserted the validity of synchronicity, a principle I applied to the sequencing of readings. I trust that you will discover more than accidental resonances in the pertinence of particular subject matter to your life at each given point in time. It may seem as if the book were reading your mind, addressing the issue or concern you most need that week for immediate application. Other times, however, where there seems to be a discrepancy, several factors may be at play. There is wisdom and utility, for instance, in taking a moment when you are feeling strongest to fortify yourself with advanced learning for a time down

5

the road when your path may wend its way back through the shadows. And vice versa, when you are feeling lost, a celebratory reading will remind you that, as the mystics report, "This too shall pass." In keeping with synchronicity, it is suggested that whatever time of year you choose to begin your cycle of readings will be the perfect point of entry for you. No need to wait for the first week of January. Start now with this week's reading and work your way through the readings week by week. Please note that some months have five weeks in some years, but not others. To make sure you are covered with a reading for every week of every year, I have included a Fifth Week Reading for every month. If you have arrived at a month that has only four weeks, consider the final reading of every month to be a bonus reading. When you've completed year two's final reading, circle back to the beginning of year one to complete your own unique transit through this perennial loop of two-year cycles.

In the end, how you incorporate this book into your life is as free and creative as your unique approach to aging. For instance, you may also want to open the book at random, trusting that you are being led to the exact reading you most need at this time. Additionally, the subject index has been specifically designed to be of immediate use to you. You are encouraged to turn to the back of the book and scan the topics to see which one calls to you, and take it from there.

This book assures you of the possibility of living life's promise one week at a time. It has come into your life at this juncture to remind you of what you already intuit: that however old you are, however challenging your circumstances, you can fulfill your life's purpose. Nothing of what you've been through, from the moment you were conceived through the present, has been wasted. In the coming pages may you discover a new level of freedom in your life that is nothing you'd anticipated but more than you'd hoped. Shall we begin?

THE READINGS

YEAR ONE

JANUARY

First Week of January

As we ring in the first week of the year, it's already time to take a break from New Year's resolutions, a simultaneously noble and misguided attempt to game the future. In the past you've invested enormous effort attempting to orchestrate the year ahead by trying to figure out which self-improvement strategy, what altered circumstance, which new protocol will guarantee safe passage through to year's end, only to realize there is no such thing. The effort, with its diminishing returns, is costing you too much. But what's the alternative?

This is the year you can instead go wild and vault into the new year with eyes wide open, hair flying. Try as you might, reality is going to have its way with you. Of course you should fix what you can, within reason; make the best possible decisions when you must. But as for the rest, you can do as the mystics teach: choose to face the future with more fascination than fear.

Just over fifty years ago, at the age of eighty-five, Jungian psychologist Florida Scott-Maxwell wrote, "We who are old know that age is more than a disability. It is an intense and varied experience. Almost beyond our capacity at times, but something to be carried high. . . . You grow more intense as you age. Inside you flame with a wild life that is almost incommunicable."

This is not the extreme sport of the extraordinary elder, meant to inspire the rest of us to take up mountain climbing at seventy or marathons at eighty. But the initiation of an even more extreme movement: that of the heart taking a leap of deep faith.

Second Week of January

Lecturing to a rapt crowd of thousands, the Dalai Lama was speaking about experiencing interconnectedness with all beings.

Olivia Ames Hoblitzelle was there and noted that as he was talking about the heart opening with the radiance of compassion he suddenly paused, interrupting his own train of thought.

"'But that's not the way things are,' he said sadly.

'We are just people groping in the dark.' And lowering his head, he began to weep openly. After a few moments he sat up, blew his nose, and continued where he'd left off."

Even our most respected spiritual leaders know that accepting not only the way things are but our own limitations can be easier said than done. Spiritual advancement does not ensure that we won't feel sad sometimes, that we won't become frustrated. But after we've had a good cry, we can simply get on with it.

When the world spins out of control, of course you should do what you can to rectify your part in things. This includes being honest about your limitations and forgiving yourself and life for being what it is and is not.

You don't have to feel happy about this, but there's a difference between feeling bad—and feeling bad about yourself.

Third Week of January

*The wistful eyes of Life are set towards
a vision that is also a Home—a Home
from which news can reach us now
and again.*

EVELYN UNDERHILL

We who have allowed ourselves to be changed by our confrontation with aging have become older, wiser, and fiercer. We regret less and appreciate more. And there are moments when we dissolve completely into a state of joy for no reason, feeling in the very marrow of our bones that all is well in the world.

But as the busyness, concerns, and challenges of life begin reaching out to grab us in again, too often it is as if nothing profound has happened.

At these times we need our poets, philosophers, and mystics to point the way back home. Home, as described by John C. Robinson, is a place of "moments of silence, stillness, and time-lessness, when it seems as if the mystery of eternity were leaking into your everyday world."

Once you have tasted this experience of merger, it is yours. Returning is not a matter of will or effort. You don't need to become more spiritual or more grounded, or to try in any way to be better or different.

This ecstatic union is not because of something you have worked to achieve, but something that comes about in all our imperfection and restlessness. As Underhill phrases it, in "the groaning and travailing of creation" you can perceive life's urge to transcend the mundane to give expression to a higher meaning and purpose.

There is nothing more to do. You are already one of us, old friend, a fellow resident of the Land of Old Souls. Sometimes we all just need to be reminded.

Fourth Week of January

Some weeks we are more aware than others of old habits, ways of thinking, and behaviors that we know are beneath us. If this is one of those weeks, the time has come to forgive yourself for still harboring self-protective, if no longer necessary, strategies of your youth that once were necessary for your survival.

For so many years you had to rely on your ego defenses—the belief that you could control things and beat the odds to succeed. Without these beliefs there would have been aspects of yourself too vulnerable to be left exposed, unprotected. However many of these coping strategies created issues of their own that you then had to address.

For instance, how often did you exhaust yourself justifying your actions when no defense was needed? How much time did you squander gathering evidence to support a fear that was never based on anything real? How often have you gone down the rabbit hole mistaking resentment for truth? At times you have judged yourself too harshly by seeking perfection, or by comparing yourself to others.

Now that you are finding the courage to set your ego defenses aside, what better use can you make of your time and spirit? Here are seven hints:

1. Relish every facet of your personality—yes, even that one.
2. Have fun, waste time, or do whatever interests you, trusting that whatever you want to do this week is as much a part of being whole as productivity, making amends, and soul-searching.
3. Appreciate that the quality of your relationships is not measured by the amount of time you spend together or degree of proximity, but by the abundance of love you carry for others in your heart.

4. Commit to living your life out of your values no matter the consequences, and even when there are unintended consequences, trust you would very well make the same choices over again.
5. Send love to body parts that no longer perform as they used to, tendering gratitude for all their years of hardworking service.
6. Accept your circumstances for what they can't help being; there are no exceptions.
7. Whatever mood you're in, whatever life has handed you, you can be kind.

Fifth Week of January
or Bonus Reading

The experience of freedom, wholeness, and fulfillment you seek grows as you continue to envision how you are going to live into your own unique experience of spiritual aging, regardless of the way circumstances play out in your life. In the higher stages of adult development you are ready to walk the fine line between holding a vision for what you really want and accommodating objective reality. This is indeed challenging—but possible.

The key to this is simple but daunting: letting go of expectation and replacing it with hope. What's the difference? Expectation has a particular end in mind. In this formulation only achievement is an acceptable outcome, with falling short experienced as failure. Expectation is inevitably an emotional roller coaster of hyper highs and abject lows.

Hope also knows what it wants and holds the space open for the possibility of manifestation, up to and including miracles. But hope rests on the solid ground of acceptance, that whatever happens is what was meant to be, and that you will be okay regardless. When hope is present, life reveals itself to you rather than makes or breaks you. In the end, when you build your vision on the solid foundation of hope, fulfillment will not be contingent upon factors that are beyond your control, and you will find your spirit to be unshakable.

FEBRUARY

First Week of February

God has come to you when you've been at your most serene moments, but God also has come to you in your darkest hours, when you were least hopeful and most unprepared.

Over time it becomes increasingly possible to remember—in both the heights and the troughs—that challenges, loss, and the many sad, bitter, and sometimes cruel faces of crises are, in fact, not impediments to the spiritual path, but stepping stones.

In his autobiography *Kaddish*, Jewish scholar Leon Wieseltier observed that, "There are circumstances that must shatter you; and if you are not shattered, then you have not understood your circumstances. . . . It is pointless to put up a fight, for a fight will blind you to the opportunity that has been presented by your misfortune."

Of course your immediate response is to steel yourself against feeling the brunt of the pain with its capacity to disassemble. No matter how many tears you shed you can't always make things go back the way they were, or the way you wished they could be. When you find yourself neck-deep in the rubble of your broken heart, how could you feel any way other than that you've failed? But the real failure, Wieseltier counsels, would be "for your heart not to break."

How, then, to summon the courage to pick up the remnants and begin again when you have suffered an anguish that cannot be willed away?

The antidote to the illusion of God as only peace is to trust that the entirety of one's journey through life is transpiring within the tender embrace of the Divine. Change, loss, and suffering are not exceptions to life. But it is also true that neither are unexpected joy, grace, awe, and acceptance exceptions, either.

And you, old friend, are called to embrace it all.

Second Week of February

This week we recommit to the real work of aging. This rewarding progression begins when we renounce our thwarted expectations that were only ever part of the false narrative that we would eventually be smart, wise, and powerful enough to master ourselves, let alone the universe.

Our expectations may not be so easily dismissed but they can, with practice, increasingly come to be witnessed rather than engaged. And regardless of our circumstances, we can tender compassion to ourselves, others, and the world, including our disappointments with how those things that trouble us the most seem to be unfolding.

As the Serenity Prayer teaches, we change what we can and accept the rest. Call it character—that mix of acceptance, courage, and perseverance that for many of us grows in tandem with the losses.

This can be the week when your sense of what you once thought you and the world were supposed to be is changed profoundly. But after the sadness you are likely to encounter something unexpected: hope grounded in reality, which is much more able to be fulfilled than the insatiable fantasies that were never real.

So this week pause to take a deep breath and consider that even if your eyes now see things you hadn't admitted to before, and even when you find yourself knee-deep in human frailty and neck-deep in turbulent times, at least you're standing.

Third Week of February

This week, celebrate that you have crossed the portal into the Land of Old Souls demarcated by the realization that things that once caused you pain or compulsion no longer carry the power to devastate.

This does not mean that things always go your way. Growing old continues to raise the bar by accelerating the quantity of new occasions to which you must arise. When you least expect it you can be shaken by your circumstances out of complacency and onto a learning curve that forces you to grow yet again through trial and error.

Of course there are still gaps, tendrils trailing from the well-worn furrows of the past in which you become entangled from time to time. But forgiveness, whether for those times you think you should have known better or for new missteps, comes more quickly and easily, and less and less do you find yourself falling into the pit of taking seriously the familiar but outgrown stories about your essential wrongness. In its stead there is a softening that gives way to what the mystics experience as a wordless apprehension of your place in the whole of things, exactly as you are.

"A door opens and I walk through without a backward glance . . . received by something far too vast to see," writes mindfulness author Danna Faulds. "'Be,' the vastness says. 'Be' without adverbs, descriptions, or qualities. Be so alive that awareness bares itself uncloaked and unadorned. Then go forth to give what you alone can give."

What is this gift you have to give? Your compassion, your hope, your gratitude. All that you've learned on this side of the door you walked through to get here. But what of when you are sad or disappointed? When you are the one suffering?

When you are fully alive there is no end to experiencing the vastness of the human potential: not just the pretty colors on the rosier end of the spectrum we would prefer, but the darker hues that younger eyes are not able to perceive. Growing old expands your capacity to see more and see with more depth. You come to realize that coupled with this expansion of consciousness is the inability to block anything. You feel it all. And then, at last, life makes sense.

And what is it you now know? That regardless of your circumstances, you're beloved. You're cared for. You're authentic. You're flawed. You're forgiven. You're grateful. There's nothing to be done but to surrender to the whole mess of it and feel the bittersweet gift of your life without feeling compelled to change a thing.

Fourth Week of February

An irony of old age is that the degree to which you fear dying is in exact proportion to how much you love being alive. Well done, old friend. You have worked hard and long to heal your relationship to life, yourself, and others, and you are succeeding. As you review your journey to the present from this vantage point, you confess that even when you did not live up to your ideals, you have never been particularly bad, nor do you respond anymore to the urge to run and rerun stories of your victimhood. They may on occasion pop into your mind, but the images—once so vivid and tenacious—simply no longer stick. You have given up feeding the lie of unworthiness that once fueled your envy, and you don't pander to the child's outgrown fear of abandonment, which does not hold up to the truth of the present moment.

Being fully alive means being open to

surprises—and when it comes right down to it, what choice do you really have? And so it is you hope that at the end you are reluctant to let go, having come at long last to love every bit of this whole crazy, challenging, wonderful, fierce experience that has comprised your unique and particular life. And then, when it is absolutely clear there's to be no turning back, that for which you hope most fiercely will not be a gracious letting go but rather a spectacular dive headfirst at the last possible second, heart wide open.

Meanwhile, why wait until the end to take the leap into the very heartbeat of life? In *The Spirituality of Age*, Robert L. Weber tells it like this: "When I was seven years old I became profoundly aware that my mother and father would die. The realization caused me to become depressed for several weeks. My mother noticed my dark mood and asked, 'What's wrong?' to which I, the scared, tough little boy said,

'Nothin'!' Finally, one day she encouraged me to tell her, and I blurted out, amid deep, deep sobs and tears, 'You're gonna die! You're gonna die!'

"She put her hand on my shoulder and assured me that, yes, she would die one day 'but, probably not for a while.' Then, slowly and quietly, she added, 'So, in the meantime, why don't you go out and play with your friends?' My mood shifted in that moment, and I did go out to play with my friends—and I have continued to do so ever since."

Fifth Week of February
or Bonus Reading

Unless this happens to be one of those blessed weeks where heaven and earth meet in your heart, you will have challenges. Some are imposed and cannot be avoided, but many are self-created, capable of being lifted by a shift in perspective.

When you are stuck in old, unwanted patterns, feeling stalled or reactive, here is a checklist of alternatives to consider:

1. If you are swept up in jealousy, try generosity instead. Jealousy is always about what you are lacking and that others have. Of course there is more you'd like to have in your life. In its positive light this is the ambition that keeps you growing, adventuring, achieving. But conversely, you can become mired in the lethargy of negativity embedded in the narcissistic belief that others have less of a right

than you to be happy. Generosity is the clear-eyed willingness to entertain the thought that you have things in your life that others would want for themselves, as well. It doesn't matter whether the generosity you bestow on others is humble or magnanimous. Generosity offers others a turn at the banquet table of life, while you give your jealousy a rest.

2. Another item on the checklist is anger—expressed or repressed. Rather than letting anger take control of you, try self-nurturing. At the base of anger is the most vulnerable part of you crying out in pain. Reminding yourself that you are worthy of love clears your vision so that if there are wrongs to be righted, you will come from an empowered rather than reactive state. Sometimes instead of lashing out, all you really need is a good cry.

3. In the midst of chaos and confusion, when you are feeling particularly sorry for yourself,

try faith. You cannot always rely on self-will to get yourself back on track. There will always be times when you've tried every trick in the book and still come up short. At these times, letting yourself hit bottom takes courage. Faith will find you wherever you are, often when you least expect it, and remind you in words already familiar to you from many sources to let go and let God. Or in the words of old soul Marika Schoenberger: "less churning things over and more turning things over."

4. While facing fear, try truth-telling. Some fears are helpful warnings, alerting you to danger ahead that you are being summoned to address. But not always. When you are triggered you are likely to catapult into the past, reliving possibilities that are no longer the potent threats they once were. Before you take action, recovery programs advise you to ask yourself if your fear is justified,

or more often than not, as they put it, just an acronym for "false. evidence. appearing. real."

5. Finally, when feeling sad, look for love. Dig deep enough and beneath the sadness you will always find love—love for someone, love for something, love for somewhere. When life gets in the way of something or someone meaningful to you, take a moment to appreciate how deeply the furrows of your love run, and have gratitude for a heart that can find beauty, however bittersweet, amid pain.

MARCH

First Week of March

This week you are reminded that even when your overworked mind argues otherwise, acceptance in the present moment is possible, regardless of how entrenched the concerns you are facing. Not to say that this isn't a challenge for those of us who learned early to start each day surveying the inner and external landscape with one question in mind: *What do I need to be anxious about today?*

For many of us, waking up in the morning is experienced less as a summons to the joy of the day than it is a call to arms. But increasingly, by God's grace, you can be taken by surprise by what is quite obvious and true: you can allow the weight of your fear-driven self-protections of the past to drag you back, or you can take a leap of faith that if you jump off the edge into a larger, if more vulnerable life, your wings will hold. It is your choice about how to live.

Must the legacy of concerns inherited from your childhood, long past, stay with you forever? Psychotherapist Robert Jingen Gunn writes that facing this question "takes us to the exact edge of life and death . . . whether to follow vitality with its attendant risks, struggles, and promise, or whether to succumb to the death within life of unconsciousness, and refuse to receive and take responsibility for that particular form of life that has been given."

It's harder on the edge where the risks and struggles of letting go are still fresh and the promise of grace is out of your hands. And yet grace comes, informing you that every moment of life is precious.

Confronted with limited horizons there is no more wasting time in emotional self-indulgence masquerading as responsibility, seriousness of purpose, or even as personal growth. There are no exceptions.

If you are confused, sit quietly until one real,

true thing emerges for you to do and then go and do it.

If there are things you need to get rid of, let them go.

If you need to enlist the support of others, let your needs be known.

If they won't help you, go get it from someone who will.

If you are feeling unworthy, be grateful for unconditional love.

This week find a moment to salute your old life and all that you constructed so assiduously and held onto so tenaciously; it has served its purpose and the time has come to release it. Goodbye and thank you.

And here's to asking yourself a new question—one that leads to freedom and full maturity: *What one thing can I do today that holds the potential for joy?*

Second Week of March

Dear old friend, we know of your many accomplishments. Did you really do all that? Where did you find the energy? How did you ever pull it all off? And, too, we know what you are capable of yet achieving. But still we ask, does this week find you digging deeper than before to manufacture the energy and motivation it takes at your age and stage of life to keep going? If so, what is it that is driving you?

Are you truly being called to perform in the same way as before, or at least to replace the magnitude of what you used to do with something comparable? Do you feel it incumbent upon you to live up to your potential? Or honestly, do you find you are motivated more by fear of who you would or would not be on the other side of all the applause, accolades, or paychecks? Perhaps you're anxious you'll be bored when the basking in accomplishment calms down? Fear that you will become invisible should the demands for you to perform recede?

This week you are older, wiser, and fiercer and have earned the right to pause to ask yourself these challenging questions. When you do you will become privy to the mystics' secret: to be old and awake is to have the freedom to choose those occasions to which you will arise.

It is up to you to decide the pace and choose the aspirations your heart dictates—that to which you are truly called. And what a surprise when you discover that even you, who have been so relentlessly busy accomplishing things for yourself, your loved ones, and the world, can find yourself on the other side of ambition with your heart still beating. Yes, even you can now just as likely be found sitting for long spells in silence, astonished to be feeling more alive than ever.

Others may misinterpret this as emptiness, but those of us who make the choice to change our pace are not devoid of anything. In fact, if anything, our hearts are overflowing. Awe, grief, joy, mystery, righteous anger, fresh insight, renewed conviction . . . each takes a turn and often they are happening all at once.

Today you are reminded that becoming whole is not something for you to accomplish or achieve. To embrace the fulfillment of your human potential you need do nothing more than feel.

Who would ever have believed that you could not only get used to it, but relish it?

Third Week of March

*To be shaken out of the ruts of ordinary
perception, to be shown for a few
timeless hours the outer and the inner
world, not as they appear to [one] . . .
obsessed with words and notions, but
as they are apprehended, directly and
unconditionally, by Mind at Large.*

ALDOUS HUXLEY

There was a time you thought of passion as a thing of the past, something that attaches itself to a flammable object, burning out quickly or smoldering over time into something often taken for granted or even becoming boring. What a surprise when you come to realize that aging can be glorious, ready to burst into love or joy or an explosion of all your senses at the least provocation.

The glimpse of the first daffodil of spring, the sensuality of walking across sheepskin with bare feet, feeling electricity passing between you and one for whom you care. Each encounter intensified with awareness of the preciousness of the moment.

You do not need to work at this feeling of being overtaken to make it happen. Aging is the elixir that thins the veil between the illusion of your separation and your merger with divine consciousness. The erosion of ego, the marginalization, the losses—all those things that you dreaded most about aging turn out to be the very means of your deliverance. Over long spans of time at last you come to understand that growing older is not something to fix or cure, but rather holds the potential to be a spiritual, even mystical, experience.

This passion, then, is the realm of conscious elders and mystics, to be held close. Something wonderful and unexpected happens with the realization that when it is your heart and not the object that catches fire, the flame endures.

Fourth Week of March

There comes a time to us all when we find ourselves sitting in peril, having encountered an occasion to which we could not rise. The one hostile exchange you could not excuse. The one request for help you knew was not yours to fulfill. The one act of disrespect you could not dismiss. But now there is a new voice whispering to you.

This is not the voice you're accustomed to, the familiar, bossy voice that you always thought was the real you. This was a voice that never whispered, let alone admitted to vulnerability. The old voice that led the charge through all the decades of your life until now could be counted on to shout from the mountaintop, "Here I am, everybody, the strong one. Take everything I've got. I'm powerful enough to meet all your needs. Have your way with me. I can take it."

Sometimes the new voice whispers, "But how many times did you deny the hit you were absorbing in the name of strength? Suppress your needs out of fear? Trade the truth of your quivering heart for bravado? Apologize for something you didn't do?"

For so long you thought you knew who you were: the one who could love until it hurt, putting the pieces back together, picking yourself up only to do it all over again. The one who could shoulder any yoke, never say no when entreated.

But now, here in the Land of Old Souls, the strange voice whispering to you of weakness and limitations that can no longer be denied has a new message for you.

"I am the voice that knows who you really are and loves you all the more for it. I am the voice that heals."

Fifth Week of March
or Bonus Reading

It's difficult not to take aging personally since, after all, growing older is happening to you. But just as young people share common age-related characteristics, whether it's a baby's colic or the mood swings of puberty, aging is also, in many ways, universal. In other words, how often do you think something is your own personal problem and it turns out to be shared by many, if not all of us?

There are the superficial inconveniences that you suffer in private. You think you're the only one with thinning hair, forgetting that there's someone else with a bald spot. There must be quite a few, otherwise why are there so many wig stores, special shampoos, and expensive treatments? And why take incontinence personally, while we're at it, when adult diapers are given as much or more shelf space as those targeted to toddlers?

Of course not all of aging's givens can be solved by a visit to the local drugstore. Illness or an accident can leave you feeling particularly singled out by fate, or even more painfully, attributed to some unwitting or even foolish action or omission on your part. In these cases statistics—even the most stark—can provide an unexpected source of comfort. How many people at your hospital are undergoing chemo today? How many in your city, state, country, the world?

Doctors, hospital personnel, and therapists will be there for you, just as they are for the thousands who have come before and even more who will come after you. To you it's a once in a lifetime experience. For them, it's what they do every day.

The only thing you should truly take personally is the voice in your heart whispering to you that when it comes to what you are facing, simply put, you're not all that special. But more to the point, neither are you alone.

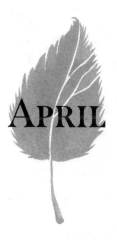

APRIL

First Week of April

This week as you review your life you will find not only one or two examples of times when you were overflowing with love, but many of them. Dig deep enough and you will know in your heart that love is love—universal, even archetypal. You'll also realize that all you've ever wanted is more love in the world.

So why is it that sometimes you become envious that other people seem to have the love you think you deserve but lack, as if love comes in a finite pot? Pause to consider another possibility. What if we all have access to the same abundant wellspring of love, which is something to be celebrated? And if that were the end of the story, we'd all be rejoicing.

But there's a hitch. The communal source of love gets filtered through the lens of each of our personalities in different ways, ranging from highly distorted to crystal clear. There are many factors, external and internal. For instance, you may have grown up in a loving family or not. And if not, you may have done the work of clearing away the debris from your original wounds or not. You may feel an easier and deeper connection to love than others who have been less fortunate or less disciplined, or perhaps your wounds are deeper than you'd ever expected and are calling more forth from you than you'd hoped.

For most of us it takes a lifetime of spiritual practice to get to the other side of one of the most tenacious character flaws—jealousy. But what if rather than envying what others have that you thought was rightfully yours, you were to aim to have as clean a filter as possible, regardless of your upbringing? What freedom to graciously tender love to others, whether reciprocated or not. What an aspiration worthy of you to view what others have through the lens of hard-won maturity, individuation, and generosity rather than distorted by competing, judging, and all the forms of ego manipulation that jealousy spawns? Turn your attention toward all you do have—the sources of love that are available and dependable, trusting that even if you do want more, all you need do is look deeper, where there is always enough.

Second Week of April

May my mind come alive today to the
invisible geography that invites me to
new frontiers, to break the dead shells
of yesterdays, to risk being disturbed
and changed. May I have the courage
today to live the life that I would love,
to postpone my dream no longer.

JOHN O'DONOHUE

Some weeks you find yourself wavering, first soaring and then descending. At the peak you feel whole and connected. This is a moment to celebrate, when you are reaping the rewards of all the hard work you've invested in aging spiritually. You've learned to let go of what you no longer want or need in your life and cherish all that remains. In this elevated space all is revealed and all is glorious. You have arrived at a place that is at once free and harmonious, full of grace and joy.

But as effortlessly as you have been lifted up, so, too, can the mood shift, sometimes seemingly out of nowhere. Slip-sliding back to the depths of the valley, it is as if you've forgotten everything. In the shadows you doubt yourself, doubt that any of the things that felt so worth celebrating just moments ago ever happened at all. Yet there exists always the possibility that the Divine will seek you out to lift you up, in whatever state you may find yourself.

In a week such as this you are called to rise above the mood of the moment and take the entire span of your life into consideration. You can see the shadows of the valleys you've traversed, the daunting mountains you've climbed, the deep waters you've navigated to have made it this far. Whether celebrating or mourning, you have been up and down often enough to come to recognize that the whole of your life is playing out against an infinite backdrop of all-encompassing love and mystery.

Embracing it all can happen to you regardless of the circumstances of your life at any given time. Even if you do not live permanently in such a state of perfect unity, once having experienced the in-breaking of the Divine, your life has already begun to pivot around this new, higher center.

If at this moment unity with the Divine feels far away, an old Irish proverb reminds us otherwise: "Heaven is always just an inch above your head." This week the call is simply to stand tall.

Third Week of April

This week we begin by acknowledging the truth that in some ways you are not who you used to be. You thought your image of yourself would go the distance, but it's cracking. And if that weren't unsettling enough, who are these poor neglected souls tumbling out through the fissures? The parts of yourself you'd thought you'd stashed neatly away long ago?

There is one who feels unlovable, another who feels unacceptable, and another who is devoid of hope. They are among the crowd of stragglers who began showing up for us when the applause stopped, the career ended, the nest emptied.

Nuisances all, they were meant to have been delegated to the deep shadows decades ago while you busied yourself building a successful life, and there they were to remain forever. The inconvenient bits of yourself were unaware of your master plan, however, and have arrived on your door stoop this week, tattered baggage in hand, asking something of you. Can you love us anyway?

It is tempting to experience their uninvited presence as a betrayal of all that you've worked so hard to construct. On these days, to assent too quickly will not be acceptance but denial. However, things begin shifting the moment you find the courage to open the door and allow them into your awareness.

When you do you discover something unexpected. For among them are not only the ones who have been let down by life, but innovators, frolickers, and eccentrics who have no interest in what others might think. This morning you will put on the kettle for all the peculiar, quirky, wounded, and disowned parts of yourself who have come, as it turns out, not to take you down but to make you whole.

Fourth Week of April

*Of all the advice in the world that you
do not want to listen to, it is the advice
of a disturbed mind.*

MICHAEL SINGER

For decades you have been seeking meaning. But not every day need be meaningful.

There are times when we are so immersed in what the week has brought for us that the voice that ponders and judges goes blessedly silent. On these days we may be deeply engaged or we may be grieving. We may simply be having fun or checked-out in quiet oblivion. But what we aren't doing is worrying whether or not it has all amounted to anything.

The truth is that it was never your job to figure out everything. When you were younger the belief that you could do so was the necessary fuel that drove your attempt to gain mastery over your life and circumstances. Did any of us succeed to the degree we'd anticipated?

Time has informed us otherwise.

Now that we are old the losses have mounted and the promise of gaining control has crumbled. To continue to throw ourselves into the rubble searching for the key when we should already know better is hubris. It is God's job to do the final summation, not ours.

Fifth Week of April
or Bonus Reading

Your willpower is admirable. How often have you set your mind to accomplishing something, and perseverance brought home the trophy? But this week's reading is for the times when willpower and persistence have failed to save the day.

Take, for example, the experience of the woman in her sixties who bumped up her exercise routine in a valiant attempt to reclaim the flat stomach in which she had always taken pride. After she had exhausted not only the available exercise regimens but herself, she turned to her doctor to request first a CT scan, then an ultrasound, and finally an MRI, certain she had a tumor. All the tests came back negative, at which point she stumbled across a box of old family photos that included pictures of her father at the same age.

Looking closely she was astonished to see that he had the same tummy bulge. Taking it in lovingly, she recalled that she had always thought it adorable that her dad hitched his pants up mere inches from his bowtie. She sifted through more photos and discovered that every aunt, uncle, and grandmother on her father's side shared the same exact silhouette. So why, when she looked at her own belly in the mirror, did she take it as a personal defeat? Thank heavens she had it in her to not only be grateful, but to laugh, finally accepting that her nemesis was not a tumor but the perfectly normal way her body had been destined to age by generations of DNA.

Perhaps the week has arrived to take another look at yourself in the mirror, not with chagrin, but with a grin.

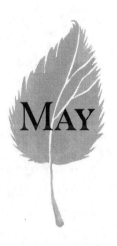

MAY

First Week of May

It is not enough to make your amends.
You need to live them.

ANONYMOUS, INSPIRED BY
THE 12-STEP RECOVERY
PROGRAM

Spiritual maturity is requiring growth on your part as you muster the courage to prepare for the future even while confronting aspects of your past that you wished you'd handled better. Of course you have done your best to make appropriate amends. Celebrate that in doing so some relationships have been repaired, some poor life choices remedied. But not all.

Our actions have consequences, some of which are unintended. You can control only your part in things, apologize for what is truly yours to own, and rectify things to the appropriate degree. But after you've done what you can to make things right, there comes the time to move on and release the past.

As theologian Joan Chittister writes: "Regret, one of the ghosts of aging, comes upon us one day dressed up like wisdom, looking profound and serious. . . . But how can it be spiritual insight to deny the good for the sake of what was not? No, regret is not insight. It is a sand trap of the soul."

You have arrived at this age and stage of your life seeking a spiritual life, a simple life. But there's an irony here as well. Rather than singing with angels, you often find yourself wrestling with them. But it is a divine wrestle, like Jacob on the banks of the Jabbok giving everything he's got to win a blessing.

Just as you need to forgive life for your disappointments, so it is that you are finding that the biggest spiritual challenge of all is forgiving yourself. To forgive yourself is to accept your imperfection. You are not especially good, but neither are you exceptionally bad. It is daunting to take on this degree of humility—to surrender to being an ordinary human being just doing your best.

In the end as you watch your illusions stripped away one by one, you accept the possibility that you may die with only one last aspiration intact: to forgive even your unintended consequences.

Second Week of May

For a society that fears aging, the go-to drug is denial. Don't want to grow old? Just don't do it. Stay in midlife as long as you can, holding onto your position and power at work and in your family just long enough to reinvent yourself into something perhaps different but just as busy and productive. This you will feel compelled to do, even if your heart is whispering to you that there must be something more.

When you were young you needed great blasts of energy because you had so many miles to go. You don't need so much now, just as much as necessary. Of course how much is deemed necessary will vary from person to person and situation to situation. The grandparents who step in to raise their children's offspring and retirees who need to find ways to supplement their income to survive are not in a position to cut back as much as they might like.

However even those who otherwise would have a choice about the intensity and pace of their lives feel societal pressure to continue to perform in high gear, stoking the fires of ambition, competitive spirit, and ego drive to stay relevant, as if they were years or even decades younger. But continuing to play a starring role in mainstream society is not a given, and in some cultures it is not a sign of successful aging, but rather of failing to fulfill one's potential as a human being.

In the Hindu system, for instance, ancient texts break the life cycle into four developmental stages. The first two stages comprise that of the student and that of the householder, active roles centering on ambition and productivity. Likewise in contemporary Western culture we are expected to excel at school, develop our talents and interests, build a career and family. But here's where we part ways from the Hindu system.

The Western models consider these years of high productivity to be the peak of human development. What comes next, if addressed at all, is at best a slow, sad decline. Where we dread the years beyond midlife as an imposed exile leading to marginalization, the ancient Hindu texts prescribe two further life stages as a highly valued progression.

The third stage is that of the forest dweller. In this vision of the life cycle one's primary role as householder and careerist gradually comes to an end. Unlike today's helicopter parents and grandparents whose lives continue to center on the family, the ancient texts considered it to be both natural and important for adult children to establish their own independent lives and to take over the active role of builders and maintainers of society as their parents withdraw from their more active phases of life.

Out of choice, drawn forward by the promise of fulfillment, the aging parents take up a simple life in the forest. In ongoing spiritual retreat, surrounded by nature, contact with one's previous life is minimal. Rather than going into town, elders are on occasion sought out by their family members and the community at large, sharing wisdom with those who visit.

But even this is not the culmination of the life cycle, for the texts describe a fourth, final stage: the renunciate. In this stage withdrawal is complete as the sole purpose becomes total devotion to God. It is in this sacred space, when you have allowed time to do its work, that you realize at last how fulfilled one can be simply taking one precious breath after another.

For those of us brave enough to explore these new life stages, the slightest breeze can be more welcome and appreciated in older age than the great blasts of energy we previously enjoyed. But this comes about only once you avail yourself of drifting through the sweet joy of the moment, no longer worrying about where you must get to or what you must accomplish.

When you experience age as culmination there is no place to go because, as the ancient texts prescribe, you are already here.

Third Week of May

*It is the infinite for which we
hunger, and we ride gladly upon
every little wave that promises to
bear us toward it.*

HAVELOCK ELLIS

Homesickness can only tug at your heart if you once actually knew a place called home. Similarly, when you yearn for connection, it is your loneliness and unrest that testify to the truth that wholeness of spirit is real and possible.

You are far more wise, loveable, and fierce than you have given yourself credit for being.

You are a precious spirit who has been called to honor what is apparent, that you have always had what it takes to have lived so fully into the present moment.

Trust yourself, trust God to guide you to your greatest good, knowing that whatever your circumstances, the healing of your heart and mind is always possible.

Embrace the depth of your yearning, understanding that you can feel this way only because you already know what merger with the Divine means, and what it is to be loved by God.

Fourth Week of May

There are mornings when, as the pitch black of the early hours dissipates into the new sun, you feel yourself tossing and turning, not quite able to cast off unsettled feelings leftover from your restless dreams. Chased by monsters, lost in a maze, exposed and ridiculed.

You may wonder if there is some message, some warning your unconscious mind is attempting to deliver to you. You may fear you have somehow gone astray, that there is some rule you've violated, there are some overdue amends to be made. But this is not necessarily accurate.

Just as likely you have encountered a forgotten aspect of your authentic self that has evaded sunlight until this propitious day. Even these discomforting aspects of your dreams come in service of increasing your consciousness.

It is a sign of your psycho-spiritual growth that this newly exposed aspect of yourself has made its way back to the surface where it can be acknowledged. You may well dislike it at first, but it should feel familiar to you since it's been smack-dab in the center of your life since the beginning. Over time it's grown bigger than you remembered and more substantial, like cardboard boxes stacked to the ceiling filled with unread books.

You could not see it in the dark, when the truth of who you really are was being chased, exposed, or accused falsely. But you can feel it now in the exquisite awakening that informs you, plain as day, that in facing up to your deeply held fears about the truth of your authentic self, flaws and all, you have not broken any laws but are breaking free.

Fifth Week of May
or Bonus Reading

Inevitably there comes a day when you wake up lethargic, cranky, anxious, or sad and don't have a clue why. Of course your first recourse is to survey the events of your life and attempt to tame the thoughts flitting through your mind. Sometimes you will find a logical explanation. You'd forgotten that your grandson has been worrying about a big exam today. Or perhaps you overdid it yesterday getting ready to receive guests. None of us welcome what we deem negative emotions, even if there is a logical, legitimate cause or explanation. On those days increased consciousness is your friend, allowing you to choose the most appropriate response.

But there are other days when you wrack your brain and still come up empty. To which the mystics reply: "So what?" One day you leap out of bed, the next day you crawl. But what if, instead of judging your mood as needing a fix or remedy, you trust your darker moods the same way you regard storm clouds? Regardless of the forecast you are not afraid the sun will never shine again. Meanwhile you can appreciate the beauty of the shadows, the excitement as the rain begins and builds, the unexpected clap of thunder. You don't always need to know why.

This week, take time to listen to the wee voice that tells you to take a day off from whatever it is you think you need to unravel. Today you need do nothing more than curl up with a good book. And if you still feel like crying, make sure the book is a sad one.

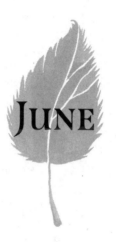

JUNE

First Week of June

You used to fear marginalization as a vast waste-land devoid of any feeling other than sadness. What a surprise this week, then, to find that even if you're alone, you're not in forced exile but have crossed into an abundant world feeling more alive than ever.

It's hard living in this new place in many ways, having left behind the masks that once offered you somewhere to hide the truth of your vulnerability. You put much of who you really are on hold for a long time because you thought that would offer you safe passage through life.

Now residing in the Land of Old Souls you are no longer able to deny the truth, the beauty, the passion of your beating heart. You see the changed world and the rubble of your outlived fantasies and feel bittersweet sadness. You hear from family and friends about the pain they're in and know you are helpless to do anything about it, but feel for them. In one beat your heart breaks, but in the next it cries itself back whole with compassion.

And there's so much more. Stripped bare you feel everything. Sitting on the river bank you merge with the ripples and eddies, only to be shaken awake with the leap of a fish. Perhaps you came to cry, but now the tears rolling down your cheeks are tears of joy.

While you are watering your plants, contentment overwhelms you seemingly for no reason. You feel the whole of your being like a puppy stretching in the sun. Then, just as suddenly, out of the blue comes a chill wind.

But where you once got swept up in anger, shame, guilt, and all the emotions you fear, the concerning feelings now sweep through you and away. With the next and every beat there's relief, self-doubt, serenity, excitement—so much happening all at once.

It can be confusing at first to be fully alive,

to have emptied yourself of protection and pretense to be in direct touch with reality. It takes some getting used to. But it can also be exhilarating, clarifying, and even triumphant, for this is what you came here for: the fulfillment of your true human potential.

Second Week of June

This week we pause to honor centenarians who take pride in their advanced age and are lighting the way ahead. The higher the number, the greater the sense of accomplishment for a job well done. But at what age did this venerable individual come to view old age as proof not only of one's mettle and good fortune but also as a celebration of a life well lived?

To answer this we have to look deeper than just the number of candles on the cake, for it won't tell you at what age she mourned the passing of her husband, when his right eye went blind, how old she was when she lost a child, the private pain he endures. Nor will it tell you at what age she saw her first bald eagle, made a new friend, or remembered the lyrics to a favorite song.

So what exactly was the age at which this person finally understood, then embraced the fierceness, the faith, the perseverance that the accumulation of life in abundance, always against the odds, represents?

Here's another question to ask yourself. How much older will you have to become before you, too, can tell yourself, job well done?

You, too, have suffered losses, taken hits, yet here you are, much wiser and fiercer than ever. So why not declare that this week is your turn to take a bow? Just look in the mirror and bask in it. So much beauty it can take your breath away.

Your eyebrows, are they disappearing? The skin on your thighs, does it sag? Is there sadness in your eyes? Are those tears of joy? You have found it in your heart to love it all and you, too, old friend, have become someone worth celebrating.

Third Week of June

Can you recall a time when you felt like you had fallen off the face of the earth into an endless, bottomless void? A place that feels hopeless without end? Are you in such a place now?

While it is true that there are moments when you know your soul is at home in the world, when the universe seems luminous with never-ending peace and joy, it is also true that you have discovered something you had not anticipated. Spirituality lived in truth is not always an ascension, but sometimes a descent.

It is in the void that you are stripped bare of your illusions, where the life you constructed but have now outgrown has the least grip on you and therefore where you are most able to let go of the past and make room for changes. It's frightening to be so exposed but because this place has become familiar to you, you no longer run from pain, from uncertainty, from fear.

You allow the breaking of denial to take with it the aspects of the status quo acquired over a lifetime that have become deadening to your spirit. And what's more, don't be shocked to discover that you do not just descend into the void once and then you're done with it. Masks that have taken decades to construct will need to be disassembled layer by layer, year after year.

But over time, emerging out of the debris of your outgrown constructions, the truth and beauty of who you truly are will grow stronger. When you recognize what has been lost you will grieve more fully. In this state when you open to the truth of your life, more will be revealed to you. Over time the pieces of a new reality more consistent with your true self will fall into place. You will find yourself enabled to look into your heart and recognize an expanded capacity for compassion, for kindness, for courage. And there is only one way to discover this renewed passion for life that does not involve falling into the void. That is to descend willingly.

"Instead of transcending the suffering . . . we move toward the turbulence and doubt. We jump into it. We slide into it. We tiptoe into it. We move toward it however we can. We explore the reality and unpredictability of insecurity and pain, and we try not to push it away," writes Buddhist teacher Pema Chodron.

This is the price to be paid for being fully alive. And this is a price you must be willing to pay. Not just this week, but whenever you are courageous enough to answer spirituality's summons to grow.

Fourth Week of June

This week, even as we transit through the Land of Old Souls, we confess we still do not particularly like aging. But we love being old and it isn't possible to get here without all the nonsense that came before it. Aging is the on-ramp but old is the arrival.

When it comes to aging we double up on our exercises and seek to reinvent ourselves. We try to tidy up all our loose ends, and they are legion. Aging is hard work. Doing everything we can to extend the illusion of mastery that defines midlife is bound to leave us cranky.

Eventually, however, there comes a day when you look in the mirror and realize that, even if it was fun, dyeing your hair purple didn't make you look younger; it just made you look old but with purple hair. And then, when you finally understand that time always wins in the end, that's when aging ends and old begins.

Old is something to be relished because unlike aging, it loves that when you trot around the living room in a dress that makes you look like a dancing bear, or go grocery shopping in your old sweat clothes, who cares?

Old loves that you've learned that when despair comes to visit, put out a tray of biscuits and she'll soon be on her way.

Old loves that you've outlasted the bullies and naysayers and have learned to stand up for yourself.

Old loves that there are people in your life who think you're incorrigible and want to spend as much time as possible with you anyway.

So here's to all of us who are aging, to those of us who are old, and especially to you who are just about to stop thinking about all this and at least for this week just live life without feeling the need to label yourself anything at all.

Fifth Week of June
or Bonus Reading

The tendency during chaotic times is to contract. When you are in reaction to what is coming at you, the spontaneous urge is to back off, letting fear make you smaller. Your heart shuts down in an attempt to self-protect, and in this state it is all too easy to turn against yourself and others.

The forces largely at play in the world in our present moment represent mass movements of individuals giving in to the shadow of unconscious reactivity. What the world needs most now is not more reactivity but more consciousness. In expanding our consciousness, individually and collectively, we make our biggest contribution and find our greatest hope.

Perhaps you feel conflicted, wondering if tending to your battered heart is really the best use of your time. Are you afraid it's selfish to take time to simply read, think, and feel? And yet despite your doubts, you have picked up this book and turned to this page for a time-out devoted to self-nurturing and broadening your perspective.

In the quiet of the present moment, right here, right now, your heart is already whispering to you that it is never a mistake to choose that which enlarges your consciousness.

Don't underestimate the importance of what you have taken upon yourself. The vital work you are doing is about choosing growth over reactivity, hope over despair, love over fear. It's about finding meaning not despite chaos, but in the midst of it.

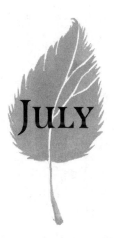

JULY

First Week of July

Over time, your experience will show
you that life, when approached with
faith—and by "faith" I mean the
willingness to surrender to reality—
won't kill you.

RAMI SHAPIRO

You arrive to this new week hoping to take full advantage of every opportunity to support life's promise: coming to understand everything that has eluded you, resolving all your life's issues, mending every relationship, and maturing spiritually. You want nothing more than culmination.

But your aspirations, even as lofty as these, deplete you and keep you busy striving at a time when what is truly called for is to make space for quiet and peace and let your life flow freely as it will.

Letting your exhaustion break you is the last thing you think you want but turns out to be exactly what you've been seeking. Give up resisting reality and at long last there comes a time when the sheer magnitude of who you really are can no longer be circumscribed by the size of your story and cracks open the container. Shards are everywhere.

You arrive at last into the realm of the awakened grownup for whom over lunch, on the phone, on long walks, the conversation has changed from complaining and confessing to intimate, familiar discoveries like sharing gratitude and burgeoning interests. Your conversations, journals, and counseling sessions are no longer filled with never-ending accusations and victimhood. Nor are you trapped in the endless loop of self-examination and self-mortification.

What can come next, if you're willing to do the courageous work of truth-telling, humility, and forgiveness and take the radical leap of faith that true spirituality asks of us: accepting that you're already good enough? That's when things get really good.

Second Week of July

Many of us feel helpless against the enormity of world affairs. Any meaningful action we consider entails some degree of risk of falling short. But life is a risk and there is no alternative.

While yours may not be a perfect action, this is to be expected, for you are an imperfect person living in an imperfect world. You can mourn this new level of confrontation with your own degree of powerlessness, but to intentionally neutralize your best if inadequate effort could lead you to a place not so much safe as fallow.

We all wish trying to make a difference was as simple as differentiating between darkness and light, but in the realms of both physics and spirituality, light is not the absence of color but includes all shades: righteous anger, disappointment, love, frustration, courage, impatience, endurance, compassion for ourselves and for human fallibility, doubt, and faith—all that goes into making us authentic and whole. And then we do what we can to make the world and ourselves better than we and the world otherwise would have been.

"This may be the hardest part of passing from older middle age into true old age: the acceptance of limits, the paring down to essentials," writes Peter Laarman. "I now think I know what the Talmud means when it says, 'You are not obliged to finish the work, but neither are you permitted to desist from it.'"

Third Week of July

You've earned the right to live life on your own terms. You are already finding yourself less and less concerned about other people's opinions, coming to realize that, as 12-step programs are fond of putting it, what others think of you is really none of your business.

There is no right or wrong way to grow old, to be sick, even to die. Claiming freedom for yourself means you get to live your life fully and freely regardless of your circumstances.

Isaac Bashevis Singer brings to life one such old soul in his novel *The Family Moskat*.

"I'm getting as old as Methuselah; I climb a single flight of stairs and my heart begins to pound like a thief's with the police after him . . ."

He goes to see Dr. Mintz who tells him to not to get himself excited. "Bad for your belly button."

"'Aha,' I tell him, 'a fine trick if you can do it. Suppose you try, doctor,' I tell him. He imagines that all I have to do is stretch out on the sofa, close my peepers, and everything is settled. That's not my way, professor. I have to roar like a lion. Do you hear me, professor? . . . I would let out such a roaring that Warsaw would collapse."

This week vow to enjoy this time of increasing freedom in your life, and not to spoil it by worrying if you are transiting this part of your journey the "right" way.

Instead give yourself permission to reclaim qualities neglected in the first half of your life, regardless of their potential for external affirmation, and to ask yourself: *What can I do that will make my own belly button roar?*

Fourth Week of July

Only people who are capable of loving
strongly can also suffer great sorrow, but
this same necessity of loving serves to
counteract their grief and heals them.

LEO TOLSTOY

When was it you last had something to mourn? Is the brunt of your losses behind you or does this week find you grieving in life's shadow?

When we are in the grasp of grief the sadness can feel overpowering. We would give anything to overcome the sorrow, the anger, the dread, and to remember the stuff of our lives that has come undone.

However, we who have already had to let go of so much have learned that grief is not an occasion to which we must rise. If you but let it, the helplessness comes to meet you exactly as you are.

There are no demands made of you, nor are there expectations.

The yarn of your life that has come unraveled will show itself to be made of strands of eternal love destined to weave themselves into new creation. But first, the way things once were must be allowed to come undone. There must come an ending.

And all the while not knowing if, when, or how this miracle will come about, the time will come to begin again, starting with the tiniest strand of hope.

Fifth Week of July
or Bonus Reading

You have proven yourself over the many decades of your life to be an excellent problem-solver. You navigated your way through childhood, figured out how to get educated, establish a career, and forged relationships, resolving the challenges of establishing an adult life for yourself. You did so by calling upon untold resources of logic and will to make it this far.

But aging is different. Inching closer to the brink of mortality week by week, you are bound to encounter challenges that defy even your best problem-solving strategies. You may try this or that for as long as you can—exercise more, get a facelift, move to a warmer climate. You may feel powerful for awhile, but eventually you are forced to admit that it's not working for you anymore. You are going to have to try something new.

And here it is. When it comes to growing old consciously, you will never succeed using even your best problem-solving tools and techniques because aging is, quite simply, not a problem to be solved. Then what is it? Aging can be a portal to an alternative universe beyond your wildest imagining. Picture a world in which other people's judgment of you rolls off your back, exacting barely even a wince for what once would have devastated. Think of what a relief it would be to know in your heart that you have more than enough regardless of your circumstances. Imagine how wonderful it would be if increased consciousness and inspired intention could at last trump reliance upon knee-jerk reactivity. What if you were to embrace the possibility that you could face your biggest fear armed only with the love in your heart? When it comes to what matters most, what if aging presents itself to you not as decline but culmination?

We seekers, sages, and mystics who have passed through the portal to old age attest to the truth that at the very moment you shift your perspective, aging is not a problem to be solved but a spiritual choice.

AUGUST

First Week of August

There are those weeks when you struggle to discern the true purpose of your life. You worry that you have blown your opportunity for greatness and there is too little time left. At these moments you feel burned out, sometimes by your efforts to inspire the world for the sake of humanity, more often by trying to get the world to do what you want it to do to make life less painful for you.

But now you have arrived at a new moment. You may be worn out from wrestling with yourself and life, yet there is a secret voice whispering to you that you are already making the contribution that is only yours to make.

You contribute every time you make the attempt to heed your higher impulses, regardless of the results you do or don't achieve. You contribute every time you shed an honest tear, surrender an illusion, or take a leap of faith.

In fact, faith loves emptiness and simplicity and rushes to fill the void with compassion. Upon this foundation of spirit you can build a better future than would otherwise have come about.

When in doubt do a little too much in the direction of emptiness and if you feel the urge to say anything at all, let it be "amen."

Second Week of August

I am astonished, disappointed, pleased with myself. I am distressed, depressed, rapturous. I am all these things at once, and cannot add up the sum. Yet there is so much that fills me: plants, animals, clouds, day and night, and the eternal in man ... a feeling of kinship with all things.

CARL JUNG

How miraculous that there comes a week when all jealousy, all regret, and all second-guessing seem unwarranted. Every insult forgiven. Every judgment suspended. When you find yourself in this new, wholly unexpected place, you can't help but want the best for everybody. Without needing to do anything about it, life makes complete and total sense.

This has come about as a result of the

abrasion of the slowly turning wheel of time that has effected the removal of all but the essential. Every incident, rejection, and complaint has been ground away to reveal the smoothed contours of what had been hidden beneath the chaos. A momentous shift, which seems so sudden but has taken the whole of your life, requires not a single adjustment of history to finally deliver long-sought joy for no particular reason.

This glimpse of essence defies reason, and while it may be the most important thing that has happened to you, is never to be found in your biography. The facts of your life are interesting, one hopes, but at least for this week, more or less irrelevant.

Third Week of August

One of the great ironies of age is that at the exact moment you most want and deserve to enjoy the serenity you have worked so hard to create, the stakes get raised. You did not expect to be saying goodbye so soon, if ever, to trusted long-term relationships. And what has become of the roles, lifestyle, and undertakings that once defined you? Then, topping it off, there's the nightly news informing you that the world as you understood it no longer exists.

It is natural that you feel each loss acutely, even as you do your best to adjust to your new circumstances. But is simply coping your best hope?

The answer can be found in the story of a man named Ishi. Ishi's ancestral home was in northern California where his Yahi tribe of North American Indians lived for generations in balance with nature. But in the early 1900s, the growing city of Oroville had encroached upon the wilds to the point that survival for his tribe had become unsustainable. Ishi suffered each loss as his people succumbed one by one to illness, starvation, and the hungry jaws of coyotes and wolves. In the end, Ishi was the last of his tribe.

Ishi had lived alone for some time when one day at dawn he walked out of the Butte County wilderness and down the streets of turn-of-the-century Oroville. Not knowing what to do with him, the townspeople put him in jail.

Before long, news of this strange appearance hit the San Francisco newspapers and attracted the attention of anthropologists Alfred Kroeber and T. T. Waterman. They brought Ishi to the University of California where he soon took up residence in the Museum of Anthropology.

Over time Ishi became more than just a subject of study. In addition to teaching toolmaking, hunting skills, and tribal stories to anthropologists and museum attendees, he was quickly taken up by San Francisco society as a celebrity, wined and dined as he lived out his days remarkably at peace with himself and his fate.

Years after they'd become close friends, Kroeber brought up something that had happened the day they first met. On that day Kroeber had taken Ishi to the train station for the trip to San Francisco. As they walked onto the platform and the steam engine approached, Ishi ran to hide behind a cottonwood tree. Kroeber then gestured for him to board and without hesitation Ishi followed.

Kroeber, after all this time, still wondered what had moved Ishi to come out from behind the tree to board the train. Ishi explained that the people in his tribe had been aware of the train but had assumed it to be a fire-breathing demon that ate people.

"How did you have the courage to get on the train if you thought it was a demon?" Kroeber asked. Ishi answered, "My life has taught me to be more curious than afraid." It seems the hardships Ishi suffered had shown him that there's no going back, only moving forward in life.

Your world, too, is changing. You find it hard to imagine how you can find it in yourself to face the challenges ahead. But you are not the same person now that you will be when your moment comes. Like Ishi, choose not to allow fear to harden your spirit, and instead grow your capacity to be surprised. When you allow your sorrow to change you, how much more curious than afraid you can become about all that lies ahead.

Fourth Week of August

Passing beyond midlife, the spiritual seeker wanted nothing more than to experience the peace she had been working so hard to achieve but that had eluded her. One summer day, frustrated and confused, she left her house to go on retreat in the forest near her home.

She entered the woods and with every step, her anticipation grew. She found the perfect clearing nestled among the oldest trees, a shady patch of green that called to her. Eager to begin, she vowed to sit quietly until God answered her. After a long time in contemplation, her mind finally quieted and her heart opened. But just then she began to itch. She tried to ignore it but the discomfort grew too intense.

It turned out that in her haste to begin, she had neglected to note that the special spot that had called to her was a thick patch of poison ivy. As the acute itching spread all over her body, she turned her complaint to God.

"God," she asked, "what did I do to deserve this? I've devoted so many years to trying to get things right. I've been good. I've been faithful. All I want is peace and what is my righteous reward: poison ivy? What could possibly be the lesson in this?"

God responded to her kindly but firmly.

"You humans. Your notion of your place in the universe is so grandiose. There was a lesson here, but not for you. This one was for the ivy."

For a moment she sat there, stunned. But then, seemingly out of nowhere, she began to laugh. She let out great peals of laughter all the way back through the forest, through her front door, and into the warm oatmeal bath she drew for herself. And as the water calmed her she found peace.

Fifth Week of August
or Bonus Reading

In the Land of Old Souls we often speak in terms of getting to a point where you can learn to fully embrace your life just as it is. But then there are those weeks when you wonder, *Who am I kidding?*

Just as surely as you remember the jubilation of crossing from the fear to the freedom of old age, there are times when you wonder if the positive attitudes you adopted about aging were real or just a rationalization. The answer is it's all real—celebration, doubt, even despair—when what it means to arrive is properly understood.

Long before you ever considered the possibility of old age as culmination, you understood all of spiritual and psychological growth to be a journey. Hard won though it was, you transited through the stages of adult development often propelled by crisis and hardship to an increasingly sophisticated understanding and appreciation of life. Taken as a whole it is becoming clear that your journey has been both a deepening and an expansion as you have carved more and more space for yourself to live the freedom of who you really are.

But in the back of your mind you always imagined a destination where all this would finally be set in stone—an ongoing state of serenity. It is not that serenity does not exist. You experienced it for yourself when you first tasted old age as the promise of fulfillment rather than decline. But what a surprise when tranquility becomes boring. What wouldn't you do for a little excitement?

Embrace life and of course you will feel low, at times, but so will you rise again, higher each time. Where you ready yourself to age gracefully, you are astonished to discover just how exhilarating old age can be. In the Land of Old Souls arrival does not mean everything is settled but that you have grown fully alive.

SEPTEMBER

First Week of September

If we had not hurt so, the psyche would have been already dead. The hurt, the suffering, is a sign that something vital is still there, awaiting our invitation to come back into the world.

JAMES HOLLIS

The fire of life can set your heart ablaze with passion, love, and hope. But it can also burn to ashes that which is most precious to you. After the blazing losses and disappointments have torn through the most painful cycles of life, give yourself time for the flames to subside.

A period of grieving is not a quick fix. It does not require tough love. This is a time for you to gently nurture yourself. Be patient. Be kind.

When the devastation feels complete, only then is it time to poke aside the charred wood, trusting that no matter how advanced the destruction there will always be one ember of life yet aglow.

When you find it, tend it with love and compassion.

Feed it with your breath.

Dress it with tender twigs of fresh fuel.

Live long enough, then someday—seemingly out of nowhere, rising like a phoenix from the ashes—you will be swept with unexpected tenderness for yourself and for others. You will feel compassion for the whole human drama in which you have sacrificed more than you had in you, and yet find yourself with more to give.

This week take time to recognize the embers of goodness, hope, and meaning that have persisted despite everything, glowing through the ashes of your suffering.

There is always an ember.

Sooner or later it will catch fire.

Second Week of September

You are a seeker. This has been a core aspect of your identity for nearly as long as you can remember. But after all these years, isn't it about time you found what you've been searching for?

There may have been decades in which your busyness distracted you, but when the tumult of midlife settled down and you had the space and time to look deeper, the old questions surfaced again. *What does it all mean? Am I truly fulfilling my purpose?*

And when aging raises the bar, as it inevitably does, *Have I missed something fundamental along the way?*

"There is no right or wrong way of growing old," wrote Ram Dass. If this is true, then why spend so much of your precious energy trying to put the right solutions in place, as though aging is entirely under your control?

Can this really be it, the culmination of your

lifelong search for answers? Can you accept this about yourself and reality, that you can never be good enough to avoid all the unwanted aspects of growing old? Can you do your best, knowing that it has always been enough without second-guessing or overthinking? Can you stand up to the officious voice that has been telling you that you can't rest until you've got it all figured out?

"We're finally free to make 'mistakes,'" says Ram Dass, to "follow our hunches, experiment boldly, or *do nothing at all*, as age liberates us from our old roles and offers us the chance to seize an authentic way of being."

So, old friend, the time has come to ask yourself the seeker's next question: *How would my experience of life be enriched if I were to take the risk of believing, flaws and all, that I've already gotten what I came here seeking?—the unconditional acceptance of my life and circumstances, knowing that without having to change a single thing about myself or reality, I am beloved.*

Third Week of September

You are right to celebrate your many breakthroughs—every risk you take that works out, every outstretched hand that is clasped by another, every fear that is overcome and crisis averted. Over and over again you have claimed new territory, lifting yourself from the shadows to the light.

But for as many times as you've managed a transition from down to up, while always welcome, may you remember that this is not the only gauge of psycho-spiritual growth. And neither is the transit from up to down, while not what you'd hoped for, necessarily regression.

The measure of true progress comes about only when you accept the whole of it and love yourself wherever you are on the cycle. Up, down. High, low. Through all the peaks and valleys of the fully lived life.

Dharma practitioner Kathleen Dowling

Singh writes: You "may have thought of the spiritual path as all-glorious, like a rose-tinged, many-petaled lotus opening into unimaginable radiance. Maybe that's so, but . . . there will be a lot of bugs and spiders and slugs that will scurry out of their hiding places in the lotus petals before those petals are fully opened."

For those times when you can experience life without judgment, recrimination, or impatience, all the while knowing you are doing even this imperfectly . . . Can you find it in your heart to celebrate this, too?

Fourth Week of September

Age is our curriculum.

CONNIE ZWEIG

How is it possible that after all these years of dedicated practice, you still can get triggered? The saints, mystics, and sages see this reactivity less as a tragedy and more as a rich opportunity for spiritual growth.

When you find yourself thinking the worst things about yourself without real evidence, much of the time it's your earliest fears that have been reactivated. Viewing your life through this distorted lens you will sincerely believe that if only you were better, different, something more or less you'd be able to fix your essential wrongness and therefore be loved.

But what if you were to embrace the possibility that reacting to old pain from time to time is an inevitable facet of the human condition and that, through no fault of your own, your early wounds will never fully heal? Then what?

Pause before taking yourself too seriously to consider the probability that when you are in this distressed state, what you believe to be the case may not be true even if it feels that way. However much you wish to remedy where you went wrong, you will never be able to cure the problem of your inherent unlovability because the truth is that you, old friend, are deeply, irrevocably beloved.

This doesn't mean there aren't real things about yourself, your life, and the world you hope to improve. But you can come to see the scolding voice passing judgment as less that of the world's consensus and more that of a petulant inner child who sometimes just needs to be treated not with a bout of self-improvement, but with a hug.

Fifth Week of September
or Bonus Reading

*Those few people who aren't a mess
are probably good for about twenty
minutes of dinner conversation.*

ANNE LAMOTT

Would you really welcome life as an ultimate culmination if everything were simply settled—as if there were nothing more to figure out, no more overcoming of challenges, recovering from setbacks, reconciling with others and with fate? While in the first flushes of spiritual aging you may feel only relief that you have found a chink in the armor of fear of growing older, it can be an equally monumental relief when you come to realize that you are still you—old patterns, unwanted behaviors, and all—and that this is something not only to accept but to cherish.

You have come a long way from the belief that your quirks and eccentricities were ever something wrong with you. Flaws are, rather, what make you so interesting. What if you were to listen to the chatter in your mind the way you take a walk with a good friend? You take turns affirming and challenging each other, always in the spirit of mutual trust. Maybe she's running old stories again. You may roll your eyes, but still you empathize. Maybe she's finally realizing something you've been trying to get through to her for a long time. You celebrate. There are times she makes you laugh, sometimes you tear up with her. Every once in a while she astonishes you with something particularly profound or especially stupid. What you rarely are with her is bored.

What, too, if the culminating life stages encompass the increased capacity to question your assumptions, to be more compassionate with yourself, to be funnier, to embrace more of the truth about life?

So ask yourself again, *Why after all these years of inner work, haven't I figured everything out yet?*—then roll your eyes, give yourself a hug, and breathe a big sigh of relief.

OCTOBER

First Week of October

By now you are well into traversing beyond the outer reaches of midlife. While some of this new terrain has become familiar to you, much remains wild territory, full of dangerous unknowns as well as wondrous possibilities. Although the task ahead at times seems daunting, this week it is time for you to congratulate yourself for making your way forward not as a victim but as an explorer.

And how far you've come! Looking back you will find it easy to recall a time when you were fraught with the challenges of growing old. Fraught is not an accidental choice of words but the most accurate way to describe a frequent mental state for much of the earlier portions of this journey. The passage from middle to older age was the hardest part: that stressful stretch of the journey where you still believed that if you just tried hard enough, you could stop the more serious effects of aging from happening to you. But only when the irreversible losses began setting in and you allowed your heart to break open did you become a candidate for serious transformation.

Happily, you persevered. You gave up the false hope of life mastery to do the challenging philosophical, religious, and spiritual work of coming to terms with the world: addressing questions of ultimate concern and the human condition, and doing the difficult therapeutic work of making peace with your past. Much of what you encountered required a greater degree of hacking through thorny brush with a duller machete than you would have preferred.

And even here, deep in the throes of your journey through wild space, there are issues of legacy to be attended to, disillusionments to be faced, amends to be made, and self-love to be administered, one act of truth-telling or forgiveness at a time. Much of this journey into the unknown has proven to be harrowing, some of it transcendent, and most of it unexpected.

The biggest surprise is that there comes a day when it all makes sense. This is the day when the fraught nature of the work is done, even while growth continues apace. You come to the culmination of one journey and the initiation of another, with time to spare.

For those who live long enough to transit beyond transition to culmination, eventually, mercifully, spiritual growth no longer centers on the metaphor of a heart broken open but rather on a heart grown whole. Congratulations, old friend, for not only have you completed your transformation from victim to explorer, but of aging from burden to cause for celebration.

Second Week of October

This week take the time to rejoice that your capacity to tell the truth, to tender yourself the respect you deserve, to live out of love not fear has grown exponentially. You have made the commitment to using your expanded awareness, coupled with free will, to respond to the Divine's call to make the best, most life-giving choice in any given circumstance.

This is no small feat, as letting go of everything that brought you this far made you vulnerable in ways you had never anticipated and did not know you could endure.

Where you were once someone who honed your skill at defending a position, you now allow yourself to doubt.

Where you once felt the need to buy love at the cost of your dignity, you are now willing to stand alone.

Where you've always been the strong one,

you have learned to receive love, help, and care from others.

And you did this all the while knowing that there is no potential for growth without risk, and that if you always knew it would turn out for you just the way you'd hoped, it was never really a risk.

Third Week of October

You know how to tender care to another, be it infant, aging parent, companion, or pet. But how are you at receiving care? For whenever life finds you in the less familiar role, here are some guidelines to help point the way.

1. Don't think of illness or injury as failure. Accepting disappointment with your circumstances is not the same as berating yourself, nor is it an occasion for self-pity. As George Bernard Shaw put it, let us determine to be "a force of nature instead of a feverish clod of ailments and grievances complaining that the world will not devote itself to making us happy."

2. If it's not part of your makeup to admit when you need help, receiving care can make you angry. Fair enough. But best keep your anger to yourself and not take it out on the caregiver who only wants the best for you.

Writes Connie Goldman, your care partner "deserves the satisfaction of knowing that their efforts made a difference."

3. Remember that you are more than your diagnosis, even if the pride you take in being a self-reliant person takes a hit.

4. Act as if you believe you are worthy of others' care. Miraculously your shame dissipates and the love that remains informs you that it is to be trusted.

5. And from Anatole Broyard: "It's important to stay in love with yourself. That's known as the will to live."

Fourth Week of October

Do you aspire to be serene about growing older, to age graciously? Think again. There are times in our lives when serenity is not what is called for, but righteous indignation.

You have learned that you have the right to live in a fairer, kinder world and to be loved unconditionally. You now know you deserve to be respected, deserve to be healthy. You have the right to stand up for yourself—to be fierce—and when life lets you down to be angry.

There will be some who prefer you passive and serene. Even when you have every right to express your raw but honest emotions, they will be quick to caution you not to overreact. When you cease working for affirmation, stop trying to ameliorate situations at your own expense, you may be told that you are in need of anger management—that you have a problem.

Of course you don't want to be an angry

person—someone who is easily riled, prone to temper tantrums and lashing out with wrath. Many of us have spent years stuffing those very feelings so as not to rock the boat, but now you can enjoy a hard-won benefit of age: the freedom to address the many ways in which you have been wronged by crying out to God that you have always deserved, and continue to deserve better.

In the Land of Old Souls there is a new voice urging you to reclaim underdeveloped parts of yourself: admitting to legitimate anger, setting boundaries, self-protecting, using your power to right a wrong.

It does not come easily at first, but speaking six little words can shiver you fully alive with the sheer passion of authentic emotion that simultaneously burns and heals, fueled by as much truth as you can stand.

"Here I am. Deal with it."

Fifth Week of October
or Bonus Reading

Who among us does not know more now than we did ten, thirty, or fifty years ago? Not just about what is right and wrong but who we are and the nature of the choices that are ours to make. Do you know more now than you did even a short while ago? Of course you do. But this week, don't answer in the affirmative too quickly for this is a trick question.

If you were to tell the whole truth, you'd have to admit to all the things you thought were true and now there is some doubt. It is actually a sign of spiritual advancement when you admit that in some important ways you actually know less now, that many things you thought you were certain of have turned out to be wrong. And an even higher state of realization comes about when there are times you feel you no longer know anything at all for sure.

For instance, you may have once thought you knew what it would entail to be a good parent and raise perfect children. You once thought you knew how to take care of yourself so that nothing much would ever go wrong. You once thought others in your family, community, even the world shared your understanding of right versus wrong.

The intrusion of reality can be unsettling, to say the least, but this can also be the initiation of new depths of character. In the place where the arrogance of youth once held sway, there is now an abundance of humility. Seeing your individual ego shatter into pieces doesn't feel good. And yet here you remain, learning not to be afraid of questioning your assumptions. Being humbled by circumstances, then, is not the abject surrender you fear it is, not evidence that you're losing it, but rather pays testimony to the fact that you've grown large enough to embrace it all.

NOVEMBER

First Week of November

There are times in our lives that call for action. Each of us has occasions to which we must arise. The problem comes when you rise to the occasion but forget to come back down again. You get into the habit of pushing through your feelings and fears, trying harder and longer, handling, managing, and doing more to get the upper hand.

It is possible that this week is one of those occasions when you must simply put your shoulder to the wheel and push through. But is this also an opportunity to ask yourself whether continuing with this line of action is simply doing more of what you already know doesn't work for you? If so, it's time to try something new.

At first glance you will probably not be all that thrilled for you will need to ask yourself: *Am I willing to pause and do something that feels counterproductive? Appear short of my potential? Disappoint others?*

Remember, you can never do enough of what you already know doesn't work. You cannot push through everything that is in your way, no matter how worthy the cause. You cannot keep draining resources you've already exhausted. So what can you do?

You can always take a longer than usual walk or pet a dog. Set an achievable goal, something that replenishes your spirit. Start small. Keep it simple. Do you have a plant that needs repotting? Is there a photo of someone you love that you've been wanting to frame?

When you stop pushing yourself to succeed and make room to receive, you set forces in motion that will bring you new insight, expanded perspective, and creativity. Before long you will find yourself overflowing with vitality, optimism, and the energy to carry out your vision. Replenished, your greatest success will come as a byproduct of the kindness you have learned to tender yourself, even when you think you have the least to offer.

Second Week of November

This week, would you rather laugh or cry at the predicaments into which you get yourself? Laughter—the adoption of a stance based on truth-telling rather than self-protection—constitutes a new adventure for those more prone to shedding tears.

Can you see the humor now in having previously thought that there is one right way of doing things to earn affirmation? That other people's needs always take priority over your own and you actually saw virtue in this? That you, above all, were the one especially chosen to fix the world?

Taking the leap from viewing life as tragedy to comedy, you can at last pack up the self-defense circus with its accompanying three rings of pretenses, and take your spot side by side with all the other well-meaning clowns, fools, and reprobates who make up the human race. And nothing of this means you can't still hope things go your way or that you can't yet do good in the world.

So if you would prefer to laugh rather than cry, this week will be easy for you. Say yes to fun, to the sweetness of life, to simplicity, to having paid your dues in full. Beyond this, everything else that goes your way will be a well-deserved bonus—an act of grace.

Whatever that was that turned your definitions of success and goodness upside down is finally losing its grip. There's nothing left for you in it. You are free to leave it behind. This is where you stop beating yourself up for failing to solve the problem of the human predicament, and instead sit yourself down and have a good laugh about it.

Third Week of November

Life is complex and the best decision is not always a simple matter of weighing and balancing the pros and cons, then doing the obvious. Sometimes when things are confused or murky you need something more to nudge you one way or the other.

So what is the deciding factor, this "something more" that tips us over to making the best decision possible?

To uncover the answer we look to a form of philosophy known as Process Theology. According to this understanding, we begin with the assumption that everything that has ever happened in the past culminates in each present moment, bringing you to this juncture where a decision needs to be made.

It is the past that got you here, but the past does not wholly determine the future because in the present moment you are free to make choices introducing completely new elements into the mix. You can make a decision that takes the greater good into consideration. Or you can make a selfish or even destructive choice. This is what is known as free will.

"Increasing the freedom of the creatures was a risky business on God's part. But it was a necessary risk if there was to be the chance for greatness," wrote theologians and philosophers John C. Cobb Jr. and Ray Griffin.

While the whole range of possible responses are present in every moment, a review of your own personal history will show you that more often than not, you made the better, life-giving choice. The question is why?

Because as Process Theology teaches us, present in every moment is the tendency for good to prevail. You already have within you intuition and wisdom that can be counted upon to provide you with the opportunity to make the choice most in keeping with Divine love.

And it is the very weight of your good intention to do the right thing that shifts the balance for the greatest possible good in your favor. This is the essential element that can always be trusted to act upon the past to create in the present moment the outcomes most expedient for your psycho-spiritual growth, just as it always has throughout the course of your life.

This week celebrate that you are free and the future is uncharted. If you but intend to do what is best in the present moment, this intention can be in and of itself the tipping point.

Fourth Week of November

*To the heartbeat of my humanity, the
tenderness of learning to walk without
hands to hold. To this gentle, most
incredible journey we are all on.*

SARAH BLONDIN

Some weeks you are more aware than others of
being radically unmoored from the past. But even
if your detachment from old ways of doing things
was self-chosen, you are probably wondering right
about now whether this is a good or bad thing.

In the past, how much effort did you invest
in fantasies that disappointed in the end? How
much time did you spend worrying about others
over whom you had no control? How often did
you damage yourself taking on problems that
weren't yours to solve?

You don't live this way anymore even though
it took nearly all you had to break free from the

outgrown patterns of loving and wounding, fixing and saving, aspiring and being disappointed that had been your habit. You did so by learning to simultaneously set boundaries to better protect yourself, and withdrawing from the misguided belief that you had it in you to do for others what they would not do for themselves. You surrendered in order to be free. But here's the truth of the matter: you may have learned how to detach but not how to feel less pain.

How humbling it is, how daunting, to accept that surrendering the illusion of control would not necessarily feel good. Your spiritual and emotional growth, while organic, hard-won, and ultimately a culmination, has come at the cost of confronting the unwelcome truth that there will always be things you don't want to happen and that you can't fix. Trading fantasy for reality represents a loss that goes right to the heart of the matter, a disappointment serious enough to require mourning. But when it comes right down to it, if you want to age consciously, what choice do you have?

Fifth Week of November or Bonus Reading

This week pause to consider those times when you've tried everything you can think of and you're still feeling blocked or triggered. You have committed to expansion with every conscious fiber of your being, but your out-of-control emotions are making you smaller and smaller. By now you've gotten stuck in old patterns so many times that you know your only recourse is to surrender and muster sufficient patience to just let it run its course. But how can you even find sufficient strength to surrender when you are feeling so helpless?

Happily, there is a formula. Do nothing to change what you're experiencing. Rather, simply describe it to yourself without judgment. For example, "I'm feeling scared I don't have what it takes;" or, "I'm tired of feeling marginalized." Then what? Whatever arises, serve as a compassionate witness to it. This is, in and of itself, growth, and of that which matters most: an expansion of consciousness.

Admittedly, viewing yourself objectively takes a leap of faith. By the very act of witnessing rather than judging you are disrupting old, familiar— even if unwanted—patterns. Without having to do anything more than this, space for that which had been blocked finds an opening.

This brings us to the second part of the formula: Be open to listening for the authentic voice that has been waiting patiently to be heard. The words need not be cataclysmic. They are unlikely to boss you around or chide you to get over it. In fact, it is more likely the words will come as a whisper assuring you that however you're feeling is okay. Stay sad, mad, or anxious for as long as it lasts, just don't turn against yourself for feeling that way.

There's a third part to the formula, and this is the only part that is truly daunting: Believe it.

DECEMBER

First Week of December

*[The spiritual life] does not take away
our loneliness; it protects and cherishes
it as a precious gift . . . an invitation
to transcend our limitations and look
beyond the boundaries of our existence.*

HENRI NOUWEN

In your elevated moments you know that expanding your consciousness requires extended periods of quiet time and contemplation. Somehow you find the courage to step outside of the outgrown busyness of your original programming, no longer willing to settle for performing a life, but venturing inward for what you really want: authenticity.

It takes time, patience, and a commitment to truth-telling to distinguish others' expectations from what you really want, reclaiming the buried and broken pieces of yourself you'd given up along the way. But there are other moments when your commitment to contemplation falters, and the distractions of everyday life taunt you with the appearance of life going on without you.

Doubting yourself and this descent, too, is an essential part of the hero's journey. Just as surely as your heart wends upward through the light of day, so must it inevitably make its way deep into the gullies where solitude creeps out of the shadows in the guise of loneliness, marginalization, and hopelessness.

Here you are reminded of the essential difference between being an outcast and being a hero, that going your own way, however it appears to others, is always a matter of choice.

Joseph Campbell, in conversation with Michael Toms, shared a passage that moved him from *La Queste del Saint Graal*, the story of the Holy Grail. King Arthur's knights were seated at his Round Table, but Arthur would not let the meal be served until an adventure had occurred. Sure enough the Grail appeared to them, veiled by a cloth. Then, abruptly, it disappeared. Arthur's nephew Gawain proposed that the knights enter the forest to pursue the Grail in order to see it unveiled, and so they set off into the trees. But there was a caveat. Each would embark on his adventure alone, following no path and entering where the forest was darkest.

Comments Campbell: "Now if there's a way or a path, it's someone else's way. People can give you clues how to fall down and how to stand up, but when to fall and when to stand, and when you are falling, and when you are standing, this only you can know."

The hero's walk requires not only the strength that initiated your journey but endurance that will hold you upright when strength falters. There are times when what you encounter requires courage you did not know you had. Threatening triggers you'd believed you'd vanquished years ago show up again—more persistent than you'd realized. On these dark days it is easy to forget that your solitude was self-chosen.

It doesn't matter if at any particular point along the way you feel hope or not. You don't even need to remember the courageous choices you made that brought you this far, nor what exactly it is that yet lures you forward. For this, old friend, is what increasing your conscious-ness looks like: not only contemplating the vul-nerability of becoming fully yourself and what it takes to grow whole, but taking the risk of living it.

Second Week of December

Isn't it a relief to be over the fantasy that love reciprocated is a given? Spiritual aging requires that you trade the romance novel's skewed take on relationship and look at your life through your own eyes. You worked hard to get to this elevated place of healing: setting and enforcing healthy boundaries without second-guessing your right to self-protect.

It has taken strength and courage to turn away from the rosy picture of what society prescribes as the good life to instead birth a free, authentic self that although imperfect, has always been good enough. This is not an assertion to be taken lightly, however. There are times when you had to face the hard truth that self-protection required you to distance yourself from others for whom you care deeply, replacing bonds of obligation, manipulation, and guilt with the freedom to grow apart, if necessary. Sometimes finding the strength and courage to let go of others felt exactly opposite from what you believed you always wanted most: what you struggled so hard to achieve, but often came up short.

All you ever really wanted was the purity of simple love, grounded in boundless trust and endless acceptance. But what those of us who grow older, wiser, and fiercer come to learn is that you don't get to merge with the kind of love one associates with the Divine without first going through the fire of being human.

You know now you can't always trust your instincts, your belief that you can try to do even more of what didn't already work and make things turn out better this time. Ironically, the fastest way through has shown itself to be to surrender to the discomforting truth you've been trying so hard to avert all of these years, which is that psycho-spiritual growth requires sacrifice.

You sacrificed plenty. You gave up victimhood, denial, and martyrdom.

You sacrificed the illusion of forced happiness to feel sadness, anger, frustration, and confusion, with no need to control or fix it. It is these authentic feelings that ultimately took you beneath the surface drama with all of its turbulence into the depths of the clean, clear water where love flows freely.

You are no longer afraid of being alone because you have already arrived to the destination God intended for you from the first: living in the sweet depths of consciousness needing nothing more, better, or different to be whole.

Third Week of December

This week as we rapidly approach the end of the year, the timing is right to take a deeper dive into the two cornerstones of spiritual aging: accepting reality for what it is, and loving yourself no matter what.

Many of this year's readings have already addressed these seminal themes and, spoiler alert, this will not be the last time you'll be revisiting these concepts over the course of this two-year cycle.

The reason we keep circling back is because there's a pretty good chance that when you read the truth about what acceptance entails, you have your own personal exceptions. You may like the idea of acceptance theoretically and would happily apply it across the board, except that you don't have the financial stability that others have so these principles may work for others but they won't work for you. Or you have physical challenges, or feel all alone in the world, or are forced to shoulder more than your fair share of responsibilities.

What you don't understand when you think this way is that we all could have some rationalization of why spiritual aging isn't going to work for us. But this is exactly what spiritual aging is calling for: that you do the heartbreaking, gut grinding work of accepting reality *as it is*. All of it. Yes, even that.

And then, while you are doing the difficult work of accepting external reality you can do the internal work of accepting everything about yourself, as well—all of your foibles, eccentricities, errors of judgment, backsliding, second-guessing. No exceptions. Period.

Spiritual aging is the finishing school for our souls, where stretching to face reality head on will inexorably lead you to the darkest corners of your psyche, the places you have longest avoided, denied, excused, explained. Here at last is what aging not only asks of you, but gives you.

Spiritual aging asks us to love life and ourselves without conditions, and in its place gives us freedom. Our circumstances may not be free. We may still feel bounded by financial limitations, physical restrictions, sadness over broken relationships, the state of the world, and all the ways we wish things had somehow worked out differently. But we do not let even these things prevent us from what we have always yearned for most: to know that we are beloved unconditionally.

If you didn't have any conditions, how could you ever come to learn this? In the act of self-accepting your conditions you are freed from interacting with the Divine transactionally, to understand that no matter what it is you have going on with you, you are valued exactly as you are and your life matters.

"Amor Fati," wrote Nietzsche. Despite living precariously on the sharp edge of life and death,

he was inspired to speak the very words we need to keep close at all times to remind us that there are no exceptions for those who aspire to age consciously: "Love your fate."

Coming to terms with your losses, limitations, character flaws, and regrets isn't easy. But for those who have the faith and the persistence, neither does any of this preclude you from making aging a culmination rather than a tragedy.

If you don't already know this, if you think you are the one exception to spiritual aging's promise, there is only one recourse. Live deeper, old friend. *Amor Fati.*

Fourth Week of December

When it comes to "Peace on earth. Goodwill to all," it is particularly challenging to find hope for the world this year. That's why it is so important today that you remind yourself that you are in the heart of the season of miracles.

By their very nature, miracles are unexpected and irrational. Miracles are not about accepting reality as it is, or even simply hoping that the status quo will work out better than expected. Miracles are about radical disruption of business as usual: not the work of man, but of a power greater than ourselves.

Yes, we still need to find the courage to change what we can, but we come to know that there are also forces larger than ourselves at work in our lives.

To believe that miracles are possible—beyond our control, understanding, and expectations— requires a leap of faith. And taking a leap of faith entails risk.

This is not feel-good spirituality, meant for happier times. This is grit-your-teeth, what do you really believe is the deepest truth about life stuff.

To be both awake and hopeful: this is the challenge. To find the courage to change what you can and believe that God can act, even when you cannot, is the true miracle of the season.

Fifth Week of December
or Bonus Reading

As you begin thinking about making resolutions for the new year, there is an important difference between giving voice to a compelling vision and fantasizing. Fantasizing is born out of denial. Lacking both roots and wings, fantasies can flip from hope to fear at the slightest breeze.

A well-grounded vision, on the other hand, springs organically out of the very fabric of your being. Such a vision is unshakable because it is not contingent on factors that are beyond your control.

This week take time to articulate your aspirations. This may be more challenging than you think. You who have passed beyond the untested innocence of youth may still acutely remember the pain that stemmed from the downside of heightened expectations. But for you who have experienced so much over the decades, the real challenge now is to refrain from being so careful with your aspirations that you shut yourself down. Being realistic doesn't mean you don't get to tell the truth of what you really want.

Make sure the vision you're capturing is compelling and authentic—both inspiring and meaningful to you. Don't worry about possible but improbable worst-case scenarios should what you want entail a risk. Understanding the shadow side of fantasy should not scare you away from having dreams. Paraphrasing Bruno Bettelheim: If you do not want to change and develop, to take risks and entertain hope, then you might as well remain asleep.

Spiritual aging inspires you to go for something you want even more than the actualization of any particular item on your list of aspirations, and it offers you the promise of fulfillment: meaning, purpose, and unconditional love, no matter the outcome. And isn't that what, at the heart of it, you really wanted all along?

THE READINGS

YEAR TWO

JANUARY

First Week of January

This can be the best year of your life, even if . . .

- You believe you love unconditionally and then a loved one doesn't do what you want.
- Despite having accepted your changing appearance, you look in the mirror and wince.
- You finally speak your truth, are willing to take the consequences, and then there are consequences.
- You've come to a place of forgiveness and find yourself setting faded photos on fire.
- Everything finally makes sense, you've healed your original wound, you believe you've fulfilled your life's purpose, and you're bored to tears.

So what can redeem the next twelve months, regardless of what it brings your way?

Hearing the voice inside you tell you that you're the only one who isn't doing spiritual aging right, and following that with your first big laugh of the year.

Second Week of January

One of the unexpected pleasures of growing older is experiencing good feelings for no reason. You relish the moment with no need to understand why or how this is happening to you. You don't need to make anything more of it; you can accept it for what it is for as long as it lasts, holding it all the while lightly, lovingly.

But as logical as it may be, it can be something of a stretch to consider the opposite: that unwanted feelings also can sweep over you for no reason.

When you feel bad you are far less prone to accept it as just one of those things to hold lightly. Instead you have been habituated over a long span of time to view a bad mood as a call to action, urging you to take it seriously, as if something were really wrong that you must fix before being able to move on.

How many journals have you filled processing an unwanted emotion only to go through the very same exercise the next time you are feeling bad? How many walks with a good friend have you taken constructing a story that may give you the illusion of a logical explanation, with the unfortunate side effect of keeping your mind spinning its wheels, stuck in false or incomplete narratives? How many times did you attempt to circumvent the crises, tragedies, and disappointments that accompany every human life before you realized you were not gaining traction but just bogging down all the more? At some point even you get tired of rerunning your complaints about the people in your life who did not love you as you felt you deserved, or whatever it is you settled on as the probable culprit for your discontent.

It takes courage to break free and resist a bad mood's search for a story, no matter how compelling the urge to regain control over your emotions. Instead, trust your soul's organic ability to process pain unconsciously. Trust your heart, your good intentions, and God. In place of the story about your heroic efforts to prevail, you come face to face with authentic emotion.

Now that you are older, wiser, and fiercer, you have learned that these emotions are no more dependable than the weather. Like a summer storm, feelings arise and quickly fade away, often from a host of factors too complex to effectively address, let alone resolve. When unwanted emotion pours down, pause to at least consider the possibility that you are not being called to solve your emotion to get to the other side as quickly as possible, but rather to hold yourself as lovingly as possible for as long as it takes.

Having learned to embrace the whole of who you really are, including the complexity of even your bad moods, you have come to understand that the true gift of life is not just a matter of controlling your emotions but of relishing being fully, passionately alive. Best of all when it is for no apparent reason.

Third Week of January

It would take a fool to overlook your many qualities. The thing is, there is no shortage of fools.

CAROL ORSBORN

Where did you get the idea that being spiritual would protect you from anything?

Yes, honing your higher aspirations has taught you much about loving unconditionally, taking better care of yourself, setting boundaries, and so much more. But when others fail to appreciate who you've become, rejecting your giving hand and open heart, or when something you've felt called to do fails to materialize, does your spirituality show itself to be unreliable?

Most of us are more than willing to let go and let God as long as what God wants for us is in the general ballpark of what we want for ourselves. If not the actual item—such as the delivery of the prayed-for diagnosis or the return of the prodigal child—at least we believe we are owed the serenity of genuine surrender and unchallenged faith.

The difficult truth is that the more practiced your spirituality grows, the subtler the urge for mastery becomes. Witnessing your spiritual essence from an elevated place can indeed bring you closer to the light, but illumination can not only reveal, but blind. When it does, the remedy is as simple as it is painful. Get real. Feel the sadness, the disappointment, the indignation, and when it's merited, shame.

But there's a caveat. When you accept anger you are still angry. Accept sadness, you are still sad. Even so you don't have to turn against yourself, thinking that if only you were working your emotions more effectively you would be happy all the time. You can be bored, grumpy, or just plain down without thinking something is wrong with you.

The irony is that yes, you are as special as you think you are. But not because of your spirituality. It's because God loves you anyway.

Fourth Week of January

In the past how many times have you taken a personal inventory of your character defects, made amends, vowed to do better, only to discover that a number of your less desirable personality traits somehow tiptoed back home while you were otherwise busily engaged in self-improvement?

You talk too much, you're too quiet, you think a lot of yourself, you're self-effacing. After all those decades trying to perfect yourself, you finally came to realize that as much progress as you've made in controlling your baser impulses, there is no right way of doing you.

Writes James Hillman: "Some of what you mean by 'force of character' is the persistence of the incorrigible anomalies, those traits you can't fix, can't hide, and can't accept. Resolutions, therapy, conversion, the heart's contrition in old age—nothing prevails against them, not even prayer."

One who learned this lesson is the great disciple Milarepa from the Kagyu lineage of the Tibetan Buddhist tradition. In this retelling of a story adapted from Pema Chodron, Milarepa is a devoted hermit, intent on spending years in solitude in a cave far above his village. His aim: to purify himself of all his attachments.

One day Milarepa left his cave to gather firewood. When he returned, demons had taken over the cave. They came by the dozens, taunting him, threatening him, and distracting him. One was reading Milarepa's book, one was in his bed. No matter how diligently he tried to keep his focus on purification, they grabbed at his attention.

Sitting in silence obviously wasn't working so he decided he had to do something about it. At first he tried to teach them about spirituality. He took a seat above them and lectured them about compassion. The demons ignored him. This made Milarepa angry so he leaped to his feet to fight them, but they just grabbed onto his arms and legs as he flailed pathetically. If he couldn't get them to leave, Milarepa decided that he had no other option than to learn to live with them.

Humbling himself, he sat down among them on the ground. At that very moment they all disappeared. All except one, which was the most menacing of all. Now completely at wit's end Milarepa thought of the only thing left to do, the only thing he could do: complete surrender. He placed his head in the demon's mouth, offering himself to the demon. At that moment the demon disappeared and Milarepa was left alone in the cave, transformed.

What Milarepa teaches us is that we can't be strong enough, smart enough, clever enough to deny the essence of who we are. Hillman writes that character is not a matter of will-power. Rather, it is character that causes you to encounter the things that happen to you in your own unique way. "This is my courage, my dignity, my integrity, my morality, and my ruin."

What a relief when you came to realize that you no longer have to deny that you are sometimes selfish, sometimes unkind. What freedom when you no longer feel the need to submit yourself to judgment or work for compliments.

After a lifetime of effort, how glorious to no longer feel compelled to compete with others or live up to expectations. You are at last unabashedly, unapologetically your authentic, peculiar, quirky self.

Fifth Week of January
or Bonus Reading

When it comes to aging our celebrity culture is doing its best to make fear of growing older a thing of the past. And how are our aging influencers going about this? By teaching us to wipe out all signs of aging and deny any of the losses associated with growing old.

Thanks to plastic surgery, weight-loss drugs, and advanced makeup products, it is now perfectly acceptable to be sixty or seventy, as long as you are a size 2 with a gorgeous head of hair. Your hair can be gray, of course—but only if it's as thick and shiny as an eighteen-year-old's. It's even okay to be eighty, as long as you are still competing in the Senior Olympics, a fashion icon, or part of a retired couple walking hand in hand through your vineyard. Fall short of any bit of this manufactured fantasy and you are bound to fret about why you don't make the grade.

The whole point of aging is to finally set your own standards and not compromise what you want for yourself primarily to earn external approval. You want to be a fashion icon? You want to run a marathon? You are in a position to enjoy a stroll through your vineyard? How wonderful—as long as it's what you really want to do. But the key to true freedom is found in the motivations for your choices. If you stop to tell the truth, you may realize how deeply societal norms influence what you believe are personal preferences.

When you fail to question your motivations you make aging more difficult than it needs to be. Shamed by the competition for acting your real age, all the while knowing you're better than caring what others think, you not only feel bad about aging, you end up feeling bad about feeling bad. But even more importantly, you are missing out on the miraculous gifts aging offers you: the opportunity for increased self-love, freedom, compassion, and individuation. This can be the moment when everything that never truly mattered most drops away and you can at last find out that you are beloved anyway.

You can't perform the way you did in the past? Can't give care to others because it is you who has the needs this time? Have you watched what you believed would be your legacy scatter to the wind? You're only going to be aging once in your life, stripped bare to your very soul. Don't miss this once-in-a-lifetime opportunity to discover that you don't need to do, be, or have anything to be beloved.

FEBRUARY

First Week of February

When was the last time you looked to see if the moon was still out in the early morning?

Have you checked to see if there's a bird flying by your window?

Does your favorite tree have snow melting off its branches?

What pictures are the clouds drawing in the sky?

When you take the time to appreciate all that you have been given, you are awestruck with life.

You've had disappointments. Of course you have. There are things you wish had worked out differently. Opportunities you've missed. Mistakes you wish you hadn't made.

But today all you have to do is look out the window to be reminded that when you've been stripped bare, the veil between your heart and the mystery is thin, indeed.

This week take advantage of this precious moment to experience the abundance of miracles that effortlessly surround you, just patiently waiting for you to notice.

Second Week of February

There is only one thing I dread: not to
be worthy of my sufferings.
FYODOR DOSTOYEVSKY

Fulfilling your potential as a conscious elder has taken confrontation of all your assumptions and coping mechanisms. You've plumbed your personal history, the depths of your soul, and encounters with reality to do everything within your power to advance to the peak of adult development.

Ironically, in breaking through, perhaps the most effective accelerants of all were the times you were faced with bad news—events that didn't meet your hopes and expectations. Disappointment. Crisis. Suffering. There eventually came one last time when you bumped up against something so big you realized you could not be good enough, powerful enough, or even spiritual enough to overcome it.

In moments of crisis you can only hope to hang onto your life as you knew it, riding through waves of panic. But even while you are crying out in pain, that which tosses you about violently is, in doing so, stripping away your old familiar roles, your coping strategies, and the hubris of your ego.

Finally the turbulence settles, the illusion of your past life mastery is in tatters, and you realize that this heartrending transit, that which you had been trying to avoid all your life, turns out to be the moment for which you were born.

This transformation does not come about without sacrifice, and sometimes you have to turn even your most cherished values upside down and your soul inside out. But what choice do you really have but to answer the summons to grow?

By answering the question posed to you by life, you discover that things are not always what they seem, often not as bright and shiny as you'd hoped. But sometimes even that which we would have preferred to avoid comes bearing the most unexpected gift: recognition of the dependable heart that has been beating beneath it all from the first.

Third Week of February

Growing old helps slow you down, limits options, provides cover for the tenderest parts of yourself. Slow is where you are grounded, nourished, whole. The recognition that you prefer to live in your small self comes late in life and is one of the most meaningful things that has ever happened to you. Digging deep into these new-found sensitivities, you find yourself capable of stopping mid-sentence, taking refuge in silence. Alone, even when others are present, you can be perfectly fine.

If you were to encounter someone while you are in this state, you may share a word, but you no longer feel the need to justify or explain your existence. You are receptive, you appreciate, you daydream.

At one time you would have judged some-one such as this uninteresting. But in this place, where living whole is purpose enough, you can look admiringly at the life teeming about you from a place that is grounded and enduring. No longer are you the hawk on a high branch poised to strike; now you are the roots of the tree.

This is not a ploy, an enhanced attempt at eliciting care or attention. The truth is more often than not that no one minds or even notices you. Nor is it anybody's business how delighted you are to be getting away with it.

Fourth Week of February

When did you start your spiritual journey in earnest? How many breakthroughs and revelations did it take to strip away the masks and illusions that separated you from divine love and forgive yourself and life for its disturbances? And more to the point, now that you're here, why are you sometimes bored?

The flatness of life without the drama has caught you by surprise. Because you have been a diligent student, spiritual aging freed you from addiction to the extreme highs and lows of your relationships and circumstances. You are neither victim nor savior, villain nor hero, but free to embrace all of it—the shadow and the light. But equanimity devoid of intensity takes some getting used to; life transpiring upon a broad horizon offering peace in place of adrenaline is unfamiliar. Does this sound like reward or punishment to you?

If the latter, now is the time to ask yourself if there is any chance you inadvertently traded addiction to the drama of your victimhood for addiction to the intensity of spiritual breakthrough. Keep this up and you may find yourself inventing problems out of habit or even just to keep yourself entertained.

How better to fill your time than revisiting old issues that once occupied you with their attendant platoons of psycho-spiritual tools, resources, and professional helpers? In place of intensity you allow self-knowledge, wisdom, and equanimity to gently permeate all of your life, not just during peak experiences.

Equanimity doesn't mean you've resolved every concern, or that you won't ever again be triggered. But you know by now that there will be light on the other side of even the darkest passages. You don't need conjured threats to generate the drama you once thought necessary for growth.

In place of intensity you ease into a place where you are free to gently experience all the good things life has to offer. Your relationship to spirituality can be about basking in the abundance of joy that requires no effort, just appreciation of the ordinary.

There comes a time when we are called to replace the challenging work of progressing through life to just living it.

Fifth Week of February
or Bonus Reading

Live long enough and you will eventually reach the stage of life informally known as, "If it's not one thing, it's another." Nobody makes it through old age untouched, and by now original complaints have spawned remedies with side effects layered beneath correctives that stack up like dominoes. Then suddenly out of the blue the fickle finger of fate flicks and the tiles go flying into what, after one crisis or another, becomes a new normal.

So what keeps the more resilient among us free-floating somewhere between peeved and intrigued, rather than stuck in despair? Here you can take inspiration from an unlikely source: Rick Steves—the travel guy.

Steves demonstrates to us how to view the unexpected bits as simply part of the journey. Whether it's a missed plane or flat tire, you take whatever arises as it comes. Then, from depths you did not know you had, you call upon patience, creativity, and grace to work with, through, or around it as best you can and chalk it all up to being part of the experience. It helps, too, if you can find it in yourself to laugh. Maybe you don't have the trip you'd planned, but what you get instead turns into the quintessential essence of the adventure of discovery that drew you to travel in the first place.

So it is with life. At some point you make a decision about how you are going to live. Are you going to wake every day in a self-protective stance, sheltering against anything that could possibly be a risk? Or are you going to venture forth through whatever life throws at you as the mystics do, trembling not with dread but fascination?

Nobody's suggesting you put yourself purposefully in harm's way. But understand, too, that bad things can happen to people who never leave their armchairs. Make your best plan, taking into consideration your current capabilities, then set forth boldly. In other words, "Rick Steves it" through whatever patch of life you're transiting, knowing that it's not all just part of the journey. It *is* the journey.

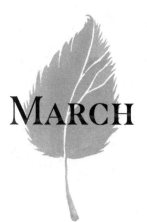

MARCH

First Week of March

Old friend, you have worked long and hard addressing your core issues. You have assembled an impressive arsenal of tools and resources to call upon when you feel bad. You have inspirational books to turn to, outside counsel to call upon, meditation and journaling practices.

And yet there are days when despite all the time and self-care you've invested, old patterns get reactivated and you feel you haven't made any progress at all.

But is this the truth?

Remember back to when you were young and your fears not only enveloped but consumed you. You didn't recognize your fear of being abandoned as an old wound, you were quite simply and pitifully sure you were unlovable.

When you gave voice to your feelings you said things like, "My life is meaningless. I've failed." Whereas now, how much more likely are you to say, "Some days I feel my life is meaningless, but the feeling will pass." It still doesn't feel good, of course, but it is not the same.

Can you remember back to the first time you thought to question what you had previously taken as truth? And then there were all the years that followed, seeking to understand, to reckon, and to rectify? And it wasn't even that long ago when you felt you had to perform for approval.

By now you know well the depth and persistence of your core issues, how early in your life they were implanted, and how vast the reservoir of your unconscious yet to be explored. Did you really think this was going to be easy?

So if you're feeling frustrated this week or disappointed with yourself, just look at how far you've progressed, that even in this sorry state you are not only victim but witness. This shift in perspective is no small thing, but the very essence of awakening.

Second Week of March

How many identities have you left behind over the course of your life? Were you once the band geek or good student, quarterback or class clown? Did you move on to identify yourself by the college you attended—or didn't complete? Where you worked? Your career or title? Were your relationships what defined you? President of the PTA? Loving spouse or disgruntled ex?

You once worried that should you leave any of your identities behind, you would be nothing. The biggest fear was that you would become invisible. But back then, when your ego was busy grieving the losses, you did not know what you know now, that invisibility can be a superpower.

Invisibility is one of the most underrated blessings of old age. How can you be judged when you aren't even seen? Wear a zebra-striped beret with sparkles and feathers. Who cares? When you are invisible you can dress how you want, do what you want, be how you want. Off others' radar, you evade definition. How wonderful when not only do you no longer allow others to define who you are, you no longer feel compelled to define yourself.

You are finally getting to live the mystic's truth: any attempt to pin you down was always too small a container for the enormity of your spirit. The sweet girl who had to squash being wild; the successful businessman who had to deny his desire to be a musician; the good soldier; the martyr. None of the roles that offered you the promise of safe passage at the cost of your freedom could ever have been large enough to encompass all of you.

In the end you burst through all the boxes, discovering that it is your freedom, not your old identities, that has always held the key to true power. You really only begin to discover what you are capable of when what others think of you is no longer your concern. Breaking out can make you brave, emotional, even demanding in ways you never before allowed yourself to be. And if you choose to be seen, God knows you can do that, too.

It is comforting to know that you no longer have to disguise any of the pieces of your essential self and that regardless of whether you are seen or not, you can live a life that defies definition. In the end, even thinking of yourself as invisible or powerful will be too small to describe the whole of who you are: unpredictable, unleashed, unrepentant, and uncontrollably, unquestionably alive.

Third Week of March

The present moment is a hologram containing every incident, challenge, and triumph that has ever happened to you. Who you are today has been informed over long spans of time by dreams and nightmares, as well as by unearned grace. Somehow you established your own trajectory and pace, all judgments about the validity of your choices proving to be temporary.

It is in this spirit that this week brings us to the portal of a life review.

Chart the timeline of the major events of your life through your childhood, the decades you invested getting an education, establishing a career, making choices about whether or how to raise a family. Who are the major players who populate the story of your life, regardless of how long or short their tenure? Recall your efforts to feel grounded, centered, safe, and loved, but at the same time, how lost and scared you often felt.

Now rerun your narrative to trace all your bolts toward increased freedom, individuation, consciousness, and meaning. At what point did your journey to safety stop being an escape from what you were trying to leave behind and a turn toward something beckoning you forward? Even when life caught up with you again, what was it about your spirit that proved to be irrepressible?

What, exactly, was the source of your drive? What was it that was always present, drawing you forward on even the slightest wisp of hope? When all felt lost, what was it that inspired you to persevere?

Crisis-by-crisis, you replaced the inauthentic bits of yourself with the self you were always meant to be.

Do you dare call this embrace of the complexity of what your life has made of you "joy"?

Yes, this is joy—joy born of surrender and acceptance, paradoxically coexisting in one heart with hope, aspiration, and pain. How exquisite this life of yours!

Fourth Week of March

There are those weeks when we worry about the future, asking ourselves if we are doomed to end up alone. But what a paradox, as this is occurring at the same time we are appreciating our solitude more than ever.

Increasingly there comes a moment when you may no longer need—or want—the complexity relationship entails. As author May Sarton once wrote, "Every meeting with another human being has been a collision . . . I feel like an inadequate machine, a machine that breaks down at crucial moments, grinds to a dreadful halt, 'won't go,' or, even worse, explodes in some innocent person's face."

Like Sarton, you sometimes crave time spent alone, actively seeking solitude, enjoying your own company, and would rather not be bothered with small talk. Of course you still enjoy friendships and companionship, but not the interactions with others that deplete you.

You are pleasantly surprised to discover just how much you enjoy your own company. At home or in nature, how could you feel alone when every tree knows your name, where the birds sing to you of their love? You are beloved by the chair that holds you, every knickknack you've collected along the way, each one bearing a memory of happiness.

What if everything were just as it was meant to be and there's nothing more to strategize, fix, compete with, or manage? What if you knew that you are already, and will always be, home, not only just a physical place where you are with particular people, but the home that is a place in your heart that can't be taken from you?

For this is the truth: Go deep enough and you realize that no matter how it may appear to others, you are beloved, connected, and whole. Friends and family may come and go as they will, but you can leave all that in God's hands trusting that somehow, in some way, just as you have enough now, so you will always have what you need most: the capacity to live fully in the center of your own life.

This is the risk that age demands we take, to look toward the future seeing yourself connected at the root, rather than getting caught up on the surface in swirls of fear. Regardless of the mood you're in right now there will be in the end a culmination—an expansion of your essence that merges with divine love. Just as you've always grown to meet the challenges fate has brought your way, so will you again.

In the meantime you are here, you are now, and you can rest assured that your deepest, quietest urge for solitude is not something you need avoid, but rather something to be cultivated.

Fifth Week of March
or Bonus Reading

Even if you are adept at keeping yourself busy, there can come pauses between projects, deadlines, or accomplishments that descend upon you with a thud. In these painful moments you may suddenly realize that when it comes to meaning, everything has come to a dead stop.

Addressing deficits of meaning, Rabbi Nathan Siegel shared this illuminating story with his congregation in San Rafael, California, nearly thirty-five years ago.

Once upon a time, a young woman wanted nothing more than to learn, what is the meaning of life? She had heard that many years ago one of the villagers had set off on a quest to discover the answer to this very question. Rumor had it that he had headed to the top of the mountain and lived in solitude all these many years. Hearing the stories, she decided to set off on her own quest: to do whatever it would take to find the old man and ask him her burning question.

It was an arduous journey to the top of the mountain, but at last she arrived. And there he was, a very old man with a long, white beard sitting at the mouth of a cave, gazing into the horizon.

"Oh sage! Oh guru!" she cried to him. "I've come all this way to ask you this one question."

"What is it, my dear?" he responded, his voice raspy from lack of use.

"Please, tell me. You've been contemplating this all your life. What, wise one, have you discovered is the meaning of life?"

She waited what seemed to her to be a very long time before the old man responded. Then, taking a deep breath, he carefully uttered three simple words: "It's the sunset."

There was another long pause after which the young woman asked, "It's the sunset?"

Then a moment of utter silence before the old man spoke again, "You mean it's not the sunset?"

Is the moral of this little story that life, then, is beyond our self-created fancies, inherently meaningless? Some philosophers believe so. But residents of the Land of Old Souls know there's something more—something that is no more illusion than gravity or electricity.

Love. But before you swoon with relief, hear this. Love is not a safe haven, nor is it an antidote to painful pauses. In fact, the more you love, the more pain you will endure.

This is one of the lessons of growing older, something you wouldn't have understood earlier in life, before aging began buffeting you about in earnest. For there is no armoring against the unwanted unknown in love, no protection from reality. And yet love is the answer to every question worth asking.

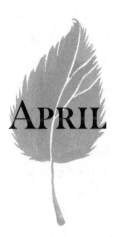

APRIL

First Week of April

William James teaches that, "There are higher and lower limits of possibilities set to each personal life." Only when we are willing to "touch our own upper limit and live in our own highest center of energy" can we hope to fulfill the spiritual potential of our lives.

This week you are tasked, as you are every week, with making the best choices possible. But this isn't always as simple as you would hope. Even the word "possible" is laden with meaning.

On one level possible asks you to dream big. What is possible when you give up beating down your spirit with busy little thoughts and bring your vital energy to create rather than protect? What is possible when you let go of old systems and structures that no longer work for you and free up your life to explore new things? What is possible when you call upon your highest aspirations and are willing to make sacrifices for the greater good?

But on a second level, possible sets a limit. What is possible given that however much you have to bring to a situation, there is only so much you can do before you must stop to refuel? What is possible given that you may be having to calculate what compromises can be made without your spirit being damaged, and what is nonnegotiable? What is possible given that while you feel called to act decisively, there are forces larger than you throwing up resistance?

If you are still confused as to what, in any given circumstance, is the best choice, stop the churning and aim, instead, to live in your highest center. There decisions are made, problems resolved as a byproduct of the expansion of your spirit into broader horizons. This, then, is the third level of possibility, where you find it within yourself to step out of the status quo and into fresh currents of wisdom previously unknown to you; where clarity awaits.

Second Week of April

In the fulfillment of life's promise nothing is ever wasted, even if along the way things sometimes feel hopeless. This is the moment to be reminded that faith often works invisibly.

Spirit is like a river flowing freely until it hits a boulder. There it pauses, piling upon itself, until the water rises high enough to push over the obstacle to the other side. The I Ching, the ancient Chinese text known as the Book of Changes, notes what you've observed for yourself, "If increase goes on unceasingly, there's bound to be a breakthrough."

When water piles up behind a dam it is invisible from the other side of the reservoir. You cannot see it rising until that one last drop carries it over the top; then there is no stopping it. Similarly spiritual practice is never wasted. Every drop contributes to raising the level. We may feel as if nothing is happening, but then, when we least expect it, life's lessons hit critical mass and push us over the top and suddenly we know things that had previously eluded us.

How many years exactly are we talking about?

As many as it takes.

But know this: despite the spans of time your faith is being tested, your second-guessing, your regressions, and your overthinking there will come a day when you will once again flow freely.

And here we pause to inquire. Why does it truly have to take so long? It's because it takes so many years to finally get past the illusions, coping strategies, and masks we once hoped would guarantee us safe passage, to instead embrace life to the fullest.

And the fact that this is a process that takes not only weeks or years but decades, this, old friend, is the evolutionary purpose of aging.

Third Week of April

What will your legacy be? Is there a university building, an endowment, or a stadium somewhere with your name on it? If not, have you at least done something significant to ensure world peace, cure a disease, or discover a new source of energy? How will you be remembered?

"Don't worry," the insistent voice in your head advises. "Even if you haven't done something on a global scale, you can at least write a letter to your adult children and grandchildren that will transform their lives by dint of your profound wisdom. Best get cracking!"

God forbid that you should take whatever spare time you can muster out of legacy-building to do something nurturing for yourself, call a friend, or have some fun.

Of course, this is not to say that if you have reparations to make to others or the world—when you have legitimate cause for remorse or guilt—you should not take the time for appropriate amends. Do what you can to make things right.

But when your work is done, how about letting what you've made of yourself overflow organically into the world in every interaction, however grand or modest? No monument. No plaque. Not even memorable last words. Let your legacy be who you are in the present moment, asking nothing in return.

Fourth Week of April

This week take time to appreciate that the part of you that used to put your own needs aside to please others has faded. Despite the fact that you were raised to believe that there is a larger-than-life, "right" way of doing things, you have grown larger still.

Having broken through to the freedom of individuation, you often find yourself so immersed in the fullness of the present moment that what others expect doesn't even occur to you. Along the way the story you've been telling about loss, fear of abandonment, and unwarranted guilt has been digested and is no longer compelling or even worth remembering at all.

Now you can recognize the rules and norms established by others for what they are and have always been: fear-driven efforts to channel, control, or deny your irrepressible spirit.

Authenticity will always be perceived as a threat by the gatekeepers of the status quo.

Sometimes efforts to contain and channel your essence were administered out of love, a misguided effort to ensure protection of the tribe. Other times the motivation was less charitable: fear or envy of your personal power. It is no small thing to claim your freedom, leave the pack, and go off on your own.

Of course there are times when listening to your own inner guidance still feels like you're violating the tribe's norms, and it's understandable that you can still catch yourself bracing for consequences. At these times it's important to remember that despite how far you've come, you are relatively new at acting from your authentic self. What novel joy to increasingly discover that because of all the work you've put into cultivating self-respect, now regret, anxiety, and fear no longer have teeth. Even the harshest judgments cast upon you more often than not slide off rather than penetrate.

Well done, old friend.

Fifth Week of April
or Bonus Reading

Age has a way of turning just about everything topsy turvy. For instance, who hasn't at some time been jealous of the famous actress who married a powerful producer who treated her like a queen? Her biography may say she's seventy, but she can still pose for photos draped in little more than the beam of a professionally aimed klieg light. Also in his seventies is the legendary athlete whose carefully curated image continues to sell everything from beer to cereal as the embodiment of eternal power.

You, too, have been successful in your own right. You may not at this moment be cruising the Italian Riviera in your own yacht, but the feeling that you really are someone is a hard habit to shake. You are justified to be grateful if fate has been kind to you—graced you with a good life, good genes, and a sense of entitlement. However, be forewarned. The more success you've had, the tighter you hold onto this persona, the more confounded and betrayed you may feel when the losses associated with aging inevitably have their way with you.

The irony is that what serves you best in old age is not your history of successes but those times when life shattered your illusions—the times you got rejected, or took a risk and it didn't pan out; the times you were disappointed, betrayed, or discouraged. You, old friend, have learned the most important lesson life has to offer: how to fail well. Unlike the famous personalities who have had the incentive and means to freeze their air-brushed personas in time—at least for a while—you have had the opportunity to learn from your mistakes, navigating your way through the treacherous terrain of broken dreams to discover that every overcome crisis has made you stronger.

What use is it to celebrate yourself only for past successes when it is past failures that have served you best when it comes to aging? How much more edifying to have discovered that life can and will tear away your masks and strip you bare, and you don't need a klieg light for your spirit to shine.

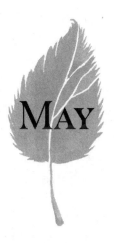

MAY

First Week of May

*This is the overwhelming, senseless
gratitude we feel when we are
finally fully awake. And it makes no
difference what we awaken to, whether
it is to pain or to pleasure, to life or to
death; it is all of a piece . . . a deep joy
when fully inhabited.*

ALAN LEW

For the longest time you wondered why you worked so hard and so long to achieve higher consciousness, yet you are still not enlightened. What is this final blockage that you need to burst through to fulfill life's promise? *The conviction that you are exceptional.*

Because you have self-chosen to carry both added responsibility and potential in this lifetime, you feel charged to be smarter, more spiritual, more whatever than others. Because you are you, the kinds of bad things that happen to others won't ever happen to you.

The truth is that as hard as you try, when it comes to controlling outcomes you don't really ever manage to get the upper hand for long. And ultimately there is no outsmarting the fact that you're only human. This, of course, is not what you'd hoped to hear when you prayed long and diligently for enlightenment, and an unvarnished dose of humility is your answer.

Behind the veil of even your most deeply held aspirations is the heart of the thing that has now stuck with you: surrender to your own fallibility, your imperfection, and above all, your humanity. You are not special in the way you'd once believed.

It is only by God's grace that at least this week, you do not feel only shame with the recognition of your hubris, but relief.

Second Week of May

This week pause to let the phases of the moon and the changes of the season wash over you. Seek out the spirals on a nautilus shell or the rings of a tree, paying special attention to a perfect symmetry beyond mere chance.

Now turn your gaze of wonder to the old woman walking hand-in-hand with her great-grandchild, each of their gently rounded tummies unrestrained by muscular strength, their wondering eyes innocent of guile, grateful to be upright and moving forward even if on unsteady feet. Child and elder both, in perfect harmony.

Is there not, then, a divine plan at play here, a sacred geometry that unites both the beginning and end of life with gratitude and diapers, unmediated emotions, and love for the moment? Symmetry in the phases of life that bring us at first out of mystery into the world, then at last back again?

So what, then, is there to fear of death? Do we not owe it the same awe, the same wonder, the same love as we tender the newborn child? Is there not a divine plan at play here, too? Nothing more to attempt to understand other than appreciation?

Thomas Merton, contemplating the end of life, wrote: "You must stop trying to adjust yourself to the fact that night will come and the work will end. So night comes. Then what? You sit in the dark. . . . It is not a matter of adjustment or of peace. It is a matter of truth, and patience, and humility."

We take this week's inspiration from the symmetry of nature, accepting that you, too, can honor wherever you are in the cycle of life and your indispensible contribution to the whole.

Third Week of May

You never enjoy the world aright till
the sea itself floweth in your veins, till
you are clothed with the heavens and
crowned with the stars.

THOMAS TRAHERNE

How wonderful now that you know you don't have to do anything to deserve to be beloved. This letting go of the engagement with the lie of your unworthiness feels counter-intuitive at first. But there comes a time when the sheer magnificence of who you really are and what you have made of your life can no longer be captured by your old story.

Acclimating yourself to this new life stage, you find you are no longer as fascinated as you once were by the hits you've taken. It's not that you don't sometimes feel you aren't being treated by life the way you deserve. But by now you've run this storyline so many times that it's become tedious—even to you. Here at the peak of the developmental pyramid, unwanted things still happen, but no longer does every transgression need be assigned a villain; nor does every disappointment trigger the need to reassert control.

When others seem to have what you wish for, you have come to realize that this is not a competition with winners and losers. Yours is now an abundant world capable of providing you with all you need, just as others get to have their heartfelt desires met, too.

From the elevated vantage point of your new life stage, you are at last getting to experience the freedom beyond knee-jerk reactivity to what is happening to you, and discover what it means to make fresh, life-affirming choices for yourself.

In the Land of Old Souls you finally understand that you are beloved not because of anything you have achieved but because *the sea flows through your veins, you are crowned with the stars,* and you are made of the very stuff of love.

Fourth Week of May

There are those days we envy the deeper connections some people have established with one another and wonder how they seem to effortlessly enjoy what we have failed to forge for ourselves. We see some family members and former friends living their lives happily enough without us, and we feel left out. But on these lonely days, are we truly estranged from others? Or are we, in fact, estranged from ourselves?

Viewed from the outside it may look as if others are getting what you think you deserve. You are stuck in an old loop, rerunning scenes from the past, present, and future seeking clues as to what else you can do to get your fair of share of love and acceptance. But how much of your judgment is based on an edited version of their lives, a romanticized narrative cobbled together to justify your self-pity?

Your wounds feel real but this pain is not

proof that you are unloved. Rather your pain is the meeting place where God's presence and your wounded spirit intersect. The greatness of your yearning attests to the depth of your love. Your longing can be a simple, bittersweet yearning that enlivens rather than disempowers.

Admit to the whole truth about your life and you won't find your sense of belonging in the showy things you covet, but in the little things that are taken for granted—everyday kindnesses, forgiveness tendered and received, unsolicited gifts, and happy memories. It is in the people who populate your life and love you for who you are, day in and out, not for what you can do for them.

Of course there are times when you want more for yourself. We all do. But you won't find it by rerunning the edited story of anybody else's life, but on your own cutting room floor.

Fifth Week of May
or Bonus Reading

How much time do you spend enjoying the outdoors? If you take walks, garden, or enjoy sitting under a tree, you already understand how enjoyable and restorative it is to spend time in nature.

But you may also be one who, while you've been hankering to go outside, can't quite find the time. All too often, even if you're retired, you've got a long list of things to do first. Everything else seems to be unavoidable, important, or necessary, but there will always be something to stop you from taking the time to self-nurture, if you let it. If not your booked calendar, it will be the wind or drizzle, and just where did you put your walking shoes? Anything will be enough to derail you.

But push through regardless and you will be rewarded with delights beyond your imagining. Has the emerald green of the first tender leaves ever been brighter? The birds, taking wing in new spring coats, more colorful?

What is old age about if not precisely for this? It may take awhile for you to realize that so much of what you've been rushing around for was never worth the sacrifice. What could life be like for you if you didn't always feel as if you have to hurry or you'll miss a deadline? If you're not always late for your appointment? If you haven't been absent-minded and double-booked engagements?

What's more, how miraculous if you knew you always had some place to go at no cost where you could remain happy or sad, anxious or floating for as long as you like, in the same way as the trees, gentle breeze, and soaring birds are occupied with doing themselves.

When it comes right down to it, "doing you" is what you do best, too. Not just important things that need to be scheduled on the calendar but being occupied fully in the midst of life, simply taking time to relish being alive.

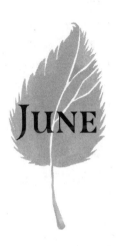

JUNE

First Week of June

*There is, apart from mere intellect,
in the make-up of every superior
human identity, . . . an intuition of
the absolute balance, in time and
space, of the whole of this multifarious,
mad chaos . . . this revel of fools, and
incredible make-believe and general
unsettledness we call* the world.

WALT WHITMAN

A time of mortal fear in the face of life and death circumstances is always the passionate present, extinguishing everyday preoccupations. It has a fierce beauty of its own, but when your ordinary fears start tiptoeing back and ultimate concerns recede, only then do you know for sure there is more life ahead of you. What a relief it is that there are weeks when you feel ordinary rather than mortal fear. You may simply feel sorry for yourself, find certain people's responses annoying, or wish you had fewer bills.

Under normal circumstances these ordinary fears, that may or may not be based on anything real, can be terrible nuisances. Sometimes they flutter through and away, other times they require processing. In all cases you believe you should be above all this already, just to do it all over again. But only if you're lucky.

Only those who have faced a potentially life-altering crisis, when ordinary bothers give way to mortal fear, can come to appreciate that the whole of life in all its resplendent messiness is to be cherished. As it turns out it is ordinary fear that is the driver behind the story of your life, without which you would be stuck in the flatlands, without a compelling narrative to play out through your good and even not-so-good choices; no breakthroughs or overcoming. At some point even the rhythmic beating of angel wings grows old and you are thrown back into the boiling cauldron we call everyday life.

So what if you will never conquer your ordinary fears, justified or not, if you come instead to appreciate them?

Second Week of June

A serious illness or accident can test our faith, but because we don't like to think about these possibilities until they are upon us, we meanwhile overlook one of the best kept secrets of old age: the transformative potential of a health crisis and the gift of recovery.

Through this lens it is possible to view the cycle of disorder and reconstitution as ritual. Pain becomes purification, loss of body parts or functions as sacrifice. In your willingness to leap the chasm of faith, you have the opportunity to leave whatever it is that is no longer essential in both your inner and outer life behind, and only bring with you that which is vital. It is a time of reassessment, self-nurturing, and reorienting around a higher center. Each breath becomes a celebration.

In recovery the dread that once kept you small and reactive loses its teeth and you find yourself thinking about what it would mean to live life knowing in your gut that there's so much less to fear than you thought. Mind you, it is possible to get this realization without first becoming ill or having a serious accident, and of course this is the preferred option. But if accident or illness should befall you, know that even this can be turned for the good.

Here, old friend, whatever your circumstances, is *Spiritual Aging*'s message to you:

You can't always stop bad things from happening.
But you can't stop the good things
from happening, either.

Third Week of June

Baron Wen Chi [a contemporary of Confucius] said that he always thought three times before he acted. When Confucius heard this, he remarked, "To think twice is quite enough."

LIN YUTANG

Something new is calling to you that cannot be denied. There are signs, synchronicities, dreams, and the welling of intuition that this is a turning point, the flipping of the page to a new chapter.

This may be an external change, such as moving to a new living situation or the initiation of an exciting relationship; or it may be internal, such as a new level of adaptation to a new normal. Whatever the nature of your transition, this represents a deepening of your spirit and an expansion of your capacity to take advantage of the propitiousness of the time.

That said, even if you know that this turning point is for the good, any change entails courage. You may be tempted to second-guess yourself, to override your gut by overthinking the possible consequences or seeking risk-free alternatives. But if taking a risk did not entail fear, courage would not be necessary.

When taking a leap of faith feels like a stretch, you can find comfort in knowing that you are supported by forces greater than yourself. This is inevitably so because it is these same forces that summoned you forward to this juncture in the first place. They would not have brought you this far to abandon you just when you need them most.

Knowing this, change, no matter how right it feels, can be at once affirming and scary.

This week, you are asked to dig deep into your heart and, in the words of Susan Jeffers, "feel the fear and do it anyway."

Fourth Week of June

Have you crossed the portal to this new week feeling the urge to reinvent yourself?

If you ask yourself whether you're truly being called to something that both inspires passion and is actionable, and the answer is yes, you should get to it. But if not, if it's a vague sense of combating your descent into irrelevance, perhaps it is time to reconsider.

Certainly none of us want to be sidelined or marginalized from fulfilling our potential against our will, so when our culture ceases to acknowledge the identities we worked so hard to establish over the course of our lives, it is understandable to want to try to replace it with something comparable.

To once again make yourself matter, the pitch goes, all you need to do is take your strengths, talents, and dreams, shuffle them into new variations of what used to work for you, and offer this repackaged self on the reinvention marketplace.

For some the old pieces will indeed be shuffled miraculously into a new and satisfying order. But for the rest of us, reinvention is not the answer. At its worst, in fact, it is the problem. Reinvention out of compulsion, not passion, steals valuable time and energy from the genuine life task beyond midlife: discovering the authentic self that has been waiting patiently for you to stop reinventing yourself and simply live your truth.

Because you are willing to take the time to cultivate within yourself qualities of character, such as patience, compassion, and clarity, you will not have to struggle to find opportunities to stretch yourself to be relevant. What you are called to do will come of its own accord and in its own time, and may look exactly the same as what you're already doing or instead like nothing you've ever imagined for yourself. The

I Ching teaches that, "When the quiet power of a man's own character is at work, the effects that are produced are right. All those who are receptive to the vibrations of such a spirit will then be influenced."

Gaea Yudron, an accomplished performer and writer who surprised herself by discovering in the midst of ambitious projects that she was in "a retiring mood," is someone who shows the way. "People will give you a lot of encouragement for doing things they consider risky or adventurous, like fitting out a gypsy wagon and wandering here and there with a one-woman show. . . . It's an overcompensation for the way our society denigrates aging, so elders are pushing to prove we are still viable, capable, worthy of notice." Yudron is content to let others carry on that tradition. "But to me, the real adventure is within: The experience of letting go and opening up to a new way of being and living. Not having to be anywhere but right here."

This week, rather than fret about making yourself relevant to others, take the opportunity to reclaim your long-denied capacity to experience life in the present moment—sitting on a park bench, spending time with a good friend, reading for the sheer pleasure—something that may not find its value in status recognition or financial reward, yet is precious beyond measure. If it's traveling the countryside in a gypsy wagon, more power to you. Empty yourself of expectations and make the space to receive. And when something catches your attention, however large or small, do it.

Fifth Week of June
or Bonus Reading

It is one of age's paradoxes that now, just when we are at the peak of life experience, we sometimes find it more challenging than ever to make decisions. For those times when your normal problem-solving techniques fall short, dive deep beneath the turbulent surface where, regardless of what you are facing, you can find resolution.

This week, your guide will be the 11-step Serenity Process. This process calls upon both logic and intuition: the whole brain and all its capabilities, topped by a big dollop of divine guidance. Above all, the efficacy of this process relies upon unvarnished truth-telling. Take your time with these questions. Write down the answers stream of consciousness or mull over each with a steaming cup of tea. The key is to simply do your best to answer them spontaneously and honestly, with as little editing and revision as possible.

The Serenity Process

Question 1. What is bothering me most? (*Don't overthink this. The first thing that pops into your mind is usually as good a place to start as any. If you don't know where to begin, just follow your thoughts, faithfully writing down every word that comes to you.*)

Question 2. What is the obstacle or challenge related to what's bothering me that I would most like to resolve right now?

Question 3. What outcome would I most like to achieve?

Question 4. How have I tried to resolve this situation so far?

Question 5. What was it about this approach that did not work?

Question 6. What can I change about this situation?

Question 7. What must I accept about this situation?

Question 8. What is my greatest fear about this situation?

Question 9. What is the truth about this situation?

Question 10. What one thing am I being called to do to get the resolution I seek?

If you would like additional input or affirmation at this point, choose from among these tools to assist you in this response. The tools are:

- Go to a favorite book, perhaps a spiritual or sacred text, and with this question in mind, open at random and begin to read.
- Pull a divination card from a favorite deck.

- Take your question for a walk in nature. As you stroll, become receptive to personally meaningful signs in the environment and pay special heed to random thoughts and feelings.

Question 11. Am I willing? If so, what's next? If not, start the process over again with your unwillingness as that which is bothering you most.

If you still don't know what you need to do, you don't want to repeat the process, or you reject the decision you feel you are being called to make: remember that sometimes the thing you are being called to do right now is to have patience and trust that the resolution you seek will come in due time. Sometimes the call is to gather more information or to let some time lapse as events continue to unfold. Regardless of the resolution you did or did not get, trust that the process is cumulative. Later today you may well find yourself suddenly knowing how to bring about the resolution that eluded you, without even resubmitting it to this process. Serenity does not only come from getting what you think you want but from trusting in the process of life as it unfolds.

JULY

First Week of July

This is a week for pausing to acknowledge the depths of your gratitude for those who have stood by you in this lifetime.

Because of them you can act courageously and with generosity, knowing you no longer believe yourself to be unlovable.

Through their eyes you have come to recognize your kindness and good intentions—the pleasure in sharing out of an abundance that is mutual.

Yes, you have walked together through many of life's passages, some smooth and sunlit, others rough and storm tossed. You have all come a long way, emerging as you did from toxic roots while aspiring to become better for it.

In each other's presence you have learned there is something more important than being happy: being real.

You discovered over time that it was possible to live without manipulating, begging, or bargaining. You felt heard and seen.

You survived conflict and misunderstandings and you no longer feel the need to resort to the hard-core drama that used to let you know you matter. In its place you are living your life as a fearless experiment, whole and free.

You have been learning partners, aspiring to experience what it means to love unconditionally.

And you succeeded.

Second Week of July

In the past when things threatened you, you asked God to intervene. But with advancing years the nature of the challenges has evolved, and God is no longer the one saving you from the struggle. God is the one calling you to struggle. A story shared in 12-step circles centers around such a critical pivot of faith.

An old woman was walking along a mountain path. The drop-off was steep but she had walked this way many times before without mishap. This time, however, a loose rock slipped beneath her foot, taking her with it over the edge.

Thinking quickly, she grabbed onto the limb of a tree as she went and hung suspended in midair. Then she felt the limb begin to crack.

This woman hadn't thought about God in a long time, but this seemed as good a time as any to resume the relationship.

"God, are you up there?"

"Yes, my daughter," God replied. "What can I do for you?"

"God, help me. Tell me what to do!"

The branch cracked a bit more. Desperate, she cried out again.

"Yes, God. Tell me!" There was a moment's silence, then God answered her.

"Let go of the branch."

"Let go of the branch?"

"Yes, my daughter. Let go of the branch."

There was another moment's silence, and then the old woman spoke again.

"Is there anybody else up there?"

Third Week of July

As you are increasingly coming to realize, nobody escapes growing old untouched. Every night the evening news announces the untimely death of yet another notable, your age or younger. Celebrities you believed to be immortal prove you can't be rich enough, good enough, famous, or even fit enough to be exempt from the human condition.

Coming into old age you will experience illness, death, and loss in your circle of friends and family. That so many have been here before gives perspective and some small comfort. But nothing can prepare you for when it will be your time to take your turn in the center of the universe as the one making the final passage.

Whatever you are facing now and well into the future, may you have faith that all is unfolding as it must and should, held within the once tender and fierce embrace of the Divine. Of course there is unfinished business, good yet to be done, words to be spoken. At times you struggle with the fear that there isn't enough time. But for this week, ask only for time enough to fulfill God's purpose for you.

In sacred time we can stop racing the clock, wasting our precious energy thinking we know better than God what is required of us. In its place we rest in life's inviolable promise that, in God's eyes, living our whole life is something we all do.

Fourth Week of July

What does loving yourself look like? You have so many lovable attributes. You can look in the mirror and see the reflection of all that is good about you. But surely by now you know some days it is easier than others. Can you also love yourself on those days when you see only flaws? When you feel unlovable and alone?

A story adapted from a talk that spiritual teacher and author James Finley gave years ago at a church in Los Angeles points the way.

Imagine that you live in a village and all your life you have aspired to climb to the peak of the neighboring mountain, where you have been assured you will find God. The journey will be long and arduous, and at last you begin.

The journey is even more challenging than you anticipated, not taking weeks or months, but years. It takes so long that by the time you are ready to make your final approach, you have grown old. You are close at last, mere steps from the peak, when you are startled by the sound of sobbing coming from the valley below you. What should you do? You are inches away from the peak, but you cannot deny the immediacy of the sorrow. Clearly you are being called.

The moment you choose to respond, you find yourself off the mountain and back in your village, following the sound of sobs through winding cobbled streets. At last you are at the source, and you realize that you have been led to the front door of your very own house. You open the door and see that there, huddled in the shadows, is a young child. You look more closely. It is not just any child; it is you. You go to provide comfort, your heart bursting with compassion as the young child gratefully accepts your hug.

"I can't always protect you," you whisper. "But I can always love you."

At that moment you look up and find, to your astonishment, that you are back on the top

271

of the mountain, still embracing the young child that is you.

As it turns out, the true test of how dependable your love is for yourself takes place not only on the happy days but when you're feeling bereft.

Your entire journey to the top of the mountain has been in service of finding God. Now that you have arrived, ask God to hold you with compassion, of course, but don't be surprised when you find that the arms God is embracing you with are your own.

Fifth Week of July
or Bonus Reading

You have questions about aging, mortality, and the future. We all do. As we confront both the possibilities and challenges of aging, the questions only accelerate and deepen. We who are so accustomed to drawing upon our wealth of internal and external resources to get answers to our questions find ourselves uncharacteristically confused or uncertain about key issues.

These are the questions that despite our best efforts persist or sometimes expand. It is as though we are suddenly in unexplored territory without a map. Sometimes this feels like freedom, at others it is just plain terrifying. But it is not that you personally don't know what the future holds. This is not some shortcoming or missed stitch on your part. None of us know.

It is natural to seek to maintain or regain mastery of our lives, but our generation is living and aging in complex times, fraught with serious concerns. The military has come up with an acronym for the nature of the era in which we're living: VUCA, meaning volatile, uncertain, complex, and ambiguous. But VUCA doesn't only aptly describe our times in general, but even in the best of circumstances, what the very act of aging entails.

The essence of this week's reading is to ask you to consider that when it comes to achieving what you say you want out of life—such qualities as fulfillment, hope, resilience, and resolution— it is the questions themselves that comprise the essence of the spiritual path. Your questions brought you here today and will serve you well for the duration of your life.

This week take particular care to honor your questions and concerns. They are not obstacles to be overcome, but the very heart of the journey to the freedom, wholeness, and fulfillment you seek.

AUGUST

First Week of August

What are you to make of those days when seemingly out of the blue you wake up feeling sad, mad, anxious, or any other of the joy-killers that hijack your brain into a maze of negativity? You may start innocently enough by asking why these worrying thoughts are in your head, seize on anything that offers an explanation, then take one dead-end after another looking for the solution.

If these don't bring about the intended result, the joy-killers stop leading the merry chase and turn to charge you with the powerful engines of your own compulsive train of thought. Before you know it you find yourself trapped in an endless loop of rumination.

Once you step on board the negativity train, every twist and turn takes you further from the clarity of the actual truth. Sometimes the fact is you don't know what's wrong, let alone how to fix it. On these days, should you choose to take your triggered mind seriously, you can easily get swept up in manufactured fear.

But then comes the day when, for the first time, you find yourself able to stop a negative thought in its tracks. Mid-thought, in something akin to a miracle, you realize that the words taking over your mind are destined to lead you nowhere, and you refuse to hop aboard. You stop yourself mid-word, halting between syllables. And you don't die.

It takes some getting used to, letting the express trains that will never take you where you want to go race past you. And how wonderful when you finally head for the station exit. You'll know which it is. It's the one marked "Joy."

Second Week of August

Did you ever sincerely believe that everyone would jump up and cheer the new you who has learned how to stand up for yourself?

It's hard saying no to bullies because your legitimate anger is mixed up with misguided compassion for them, and your efforts at boundary-setting are undermined by guilt for whatever role you've played in the past, accepting that you're the "cause" of others' unhappiness. Yes, you may have contributed, but do you bear complete responsibility? Becoming whole will require letting go of the remorseful story you've been telling everybody, forgiving yourself and learning to self-protect. You may not be perfect, but even imperfect human beings have rights.

This is no less than a complete renovation, facing down your fear of exile from the tribe, getting to a place where there is nothing left to prove or achieve. Self-love is key but is no inoculation against the fact that things may still go awry.

Now is the time to ask yourself which voice is worthy of you. The one that proclaims you deserve respect? Or the one that whimpers you deserve what you got? You know which one has your best interests at heart, even if paying heed to it is likely to cost you something.

Third Week of August

In the past you have been on the run from the enormity of the world's problems, chased by the fear of falling short. The task ahead is daunting, too big for one person.

And yet the time has come to stop running and take a stand. You must do what is yours to do.

The moment you begin acting as if your frustration is not about your inadequacy but rather about that which yearns to grow larger, the fearsome forces that have been pushing you from behind give way.

Where to begin?

There is always only one place. Find the courage to live out of your values, no matter how it may turn out, by simply making one good choice at a time.

Choose to break the hubris of control and surrender to humility and you will see things more clearly. When you take action you will be motivated by love, not the will to power over others.

Expand your perspective and you will discover that you can be patient and passionate, kind and fierce. Even when it seems to be almost more than you can bear, you can continue to hope and try your best to bring more consciousness into a world that needs its wise elders now more than ever.

If this is the occasion to which you must arise, hear this: how you choose to respond matters. It may not seem to you to be enough, but it is everything.

Fourth Week of August

One must affirm one's own destiny,
play the cards one has been dealt, for
this is how we forge an ego that does
not break down under duress.

CARL JUNG

When you commit yourself to the path of spiritual aging, you learn something important about what it means to be resilient. Resilience is not a heroic struggle with life's challenges to return things to the way they were and emerge unaltered. Rather, resilience is the call to rise to life's many occasions, allowing yourself to be changed by them.

You must surrender even your most cherished notions of what it means to be powerful, to be successful, to overcome all obstacles. In its place you will discover new depths to your capacity for vulnerability, humility, and compassion. You will feel more.

In the upside-down world of spiritual progress, to aim to overcome all obstacles to fulfill life's promise is not proof of your sincere desire to do what life asks of you, but grandiosity. Here in the Land of Old Souls you are summoned to play the hand you've been dealt with as much consciousness as you can muster.

For Carl Jung the very purpose of life was this passionate urge for deeper understanding: "Not the players or events of your life but what you've made of them in terms of increasing your consciousness."

So, old friend, if you are conscious of having made mistakes, of losing control, of falling short of protecting yourself and those for whom you care, you are not only on the right track, but in good company. At this point the cutting edge of your learning will not be to wish to have done life perfectly, but to cut yourself slack.

Consciousness, Jung teaches, not perfection, is the path to meaning.

Fifth Week of August
or Bonus Reading

*The familiar life horizon has been
outgrown; the old concepts, ideals,
and emotional patterns no longer fit;
the time for the passing of a threshold
is at hand.*

JOSEPH CAMPBELL

What aspects of yourself did you neglect in the
first half of your life that you are now free to
develop? This week is an opportunity for you to
go even deeper, questioning conceptions you've
been holding, often unconsciously, of whom you
thought you were, in order to reenergize your
understanding of what it means to grow into
your authentic self.

Becoming increasingly authentic does not
mean leaving behind everything you brought
to this present moment. You may discover that

there are aspects and qualities about yourself that you want to retain, expand, or deepen. Of course there are. But you may also discover something unexpected, that this precious moment of time is an opportunity to explore new ways of relating to the world. In fact, many who have mastered certain ways of being are curious and eager to experience the exact flipside, at least for a short time.

The flipside is different for everyone. Someone who has always been quiet and supportive of others may want to experience what it's like to be the center of attention and feel powerful, for a change. On the other hand, someone who has already mastered being powerful and gathering attention may crave solitude and anonymity.

Over time most return to retrieve some of what they had thought to leave behind forever in order to meld together something authentic, original, and unshakable. This is the essence of what many of us say we want most out of life, for the key to consciously aging, as Connie Goldman was fond of saying, is to aspire to not only grow old, but to grow whole.

SEPTEMBER

First Week of September

How many hours, years, decades have you devoted yourself to taking on problems that were never yours to solve in the first place? You have always been diligent, but now you are also experienced and know better.

What's weighing on your mind right now? If you were to pause at the first moment a concern enters your mind, you would already know where your line of thinking will lead. Is there the potential for a resolution that will be worth your investment of time and energy? Or are you indulging yourself with useless churning over things that you can't, won't, or shouldn't take on? And then, too, will your well-meaning but misguided efforts spill over to others in the form of meddling, dumping, or disrespect?

If the problem is new or ripe, of course, it is important to take the time to think it through, and if there's something that occurs to you that could positively affect the outcome, do it. But if you bring your best thinking to it to no avail—or if what's bothering you is old, familiar, or persistent—don't waste one second more of your precious life looking for solutions your heart knows you won't find. The descent into worrying, fretting, and overworking problems can be aborted the moment you trade thinking it through for truth-telling.

If it's time to let go, it's not that you won't be sad or frustrated or humbled. But these are emotions, not thoughts—the very thing all that thinking was working overtime to avoid. If admitting there is nothing more you can do is cause for grief, grief it is. The end to fruitless worrying is found in your heart, not your head.

Trust the truth, trust your heart, and in the end, come what may, you can take comfort in knowing you have done everything in your power to bring about the best outcome possible.

Second Week of September

Of course you want to do what you can to live your best possible life. But when it comes to the particular challenge at hand, do you sometimes find yourself wondering which is the right thing to do: push through the obstacle or accept what is?

If you listen to the heroic voice of the warrior within, you'll be warned that surrender is always premature. "You're weak if you stop fighting too soon. Never give up hope." Cue the triumphant music because no matter how tired you are, how bleak the prognosis, you've got what it takes. And often you do.

But there are other times when in your heart of hearts, try as hard as you might, there are no magic arrows in your quiver. You could keep fighting at least for awhile if you want, but why? Not every occasion calls upon you to play the hero. You don't always need to go to great lengths, try harder, learn more, or do anything at all if you surrender to the divine love guiding you to accept your life as it is.

You, old friend, already live here. You know this. But the worn-out warrior who has been struggling all those years to get you here doesn't recognize that you have arrived.

When you are faced with a challenge and you feel called to rise to the occasion, Godspeed! But consider, too, how early this is in your process of casting off the old heroic models; how little experience you have in accepting the divine love that is already promised.

Whatever you choose, do so trusting that you are already in the embrace of a deep love that goes to the very root of divine consciousness. There are no mistakes here, only the fulfillment of life's promise, whatever it is you choose.

Third Week of September

This week, as most weeks, you are aware that there is distance between the way you wish things were—both for yourself and for the world—and what is.

Through good times and bad we humans yearn for merger with the Divine. But so much of life is spent trying to manage the pieces flying at us, broken only by the occasional transcendent moment while doing t'ai chi or watching a particularly resplendent sunrise. We get the dishes washed. We file our tax returns. We have our routines and what we consider to be "normal," which is often pleasurable enough, other times dull and alienating. We persevere and hope there's no more bad news on its way.

But all this begs the question: What if, as long as we are alive and things keep happening to us and the world, we never achieve the ongoing merger with the Divine for which we strive?

The truth is that we are all limited, finite, mortal, human. The original wound is universal and inevitable, and everything that subsequently unfolds throughout the many stages of our lives is not just personal.

You remedy what you can, of course. And happily there are some things that are under your control. But not all. For instance, you are not to judge yourself as guilty for actions for which you intended good but that went woefully awry. You can't make amends for what is not yours to fix. Not for what is in your DNA, archetypal forces, anybody else's choices, or the 96 percent of your brain that scientists postulate is unconscious. Nor can you change how others feel about who you are when you become less willing to compromise, hide, or defend your true self. Once you have rectified all that you can, there can still be sadness or disappointment but there is no more cause for guilt. And yet, the gap between what you hope for and reality persists.

Here, then, arrives a second, equally provocative question for you to ponder: But what if this is not failure? For it is in the gap between reality and aspiration that creativity arises. In the breech is where we explore, experiment, practice, and build. In the gap we are humbled, vulnerable, worn down to a nub of authenticity. In the gap there are times, as well, when we simply endure. But even this implies some lure drawing us forward toward hope, however dimly felt.

Is the gap, then, the source of meaning and of purpose, where you are called to aspire to something akin to greatness? Is heeding the call for merger with the Divine not exclusively the point of life but rather a foretaste of things to come? And in the meanwhile, life is sometimes peaceful, sometimes upsetting, sometimes dull. But however disappointing life may be at any given time, one thing is for sure: you want more.

Fourth Week of September

Does this week find you asking yourself, *Am I doing enough to make this world a better place?* Take courage in knowing that it is better to wrestle with the question than settle for superficial resolution. The very fact of your honest discomfort is a good sign that you are up to the task of doing your share.

Faced with the enormity of the world's pain, it is all too easy to seek premature refuge in the name of spirituality. Some who believe they are withholding judgment out of compassion or tolerance may have inadvertently become complicit. Acceptance, when misunderstood, can be confused with complacency or even the normalization of evil. Aspiring to find peace is honorable but can lead some to mistake serenity for what is, in reality, hiding—and for others a cover for self-righteousness.

Genuine faith asks the impossible of you: to

trust that all will be well. But not on your time-table, or in the way you would prefer, and not necessarily without discomfort.

Facing your limitations in view of the weight of the world's pain does not excuse you from right action, but ensures that when you do act, you will not have muddied your connection to God with impatience, grandiosity, self-pity, or the exhausting struggle to wrest control.

Sober, loving, honest, imperfect, in pain (or not), ask yourself again: *Am I doing enough?* Here's your answer: *When my heart calls to me, will I abide?*

Fifth Week of September
or Bonus Reading

This week take the opportunity to give a hearty shout-out to the good boy or girl you once were, the child who worked hard to please others, and whom you thought you'd left behind long ago. You have gone through so many life stages since you were a baby, from utter dependence to individuation.

As a child you sought approval. In your teens you rebelled. At midlife you reinvented yourself. Beyond your middle years you have worked long and hard to recover your authentic voice, to discover who you are apart from early influences. It's been a long, long time since your primary concern has been to fit in: to not rock any boats and therefore be affirmed by the tribe. You thought you were finished with requiring validation.

So, then, why on earth do you ever spend a single second of your precious time seeking approval for the way you're aging? Do you find yourself scanning the horizon to assess how you're aging in comparison to others? Do you feel a twinge in the presence of someone your age who is closer to their children, has more savings, fewer wrinkles, or is in better health, as if any of these is some objective gauge by which to measure yourself? Wherever did you get the outlandish idea that there is a right and wrong way to grow older?

If you are mortified that at this advanced age and stage of life you are in some ways still seeking external validation, this is a good thing. Remember that telling the truth, even if uncomfortable, is the cornerstone of spiritual aging. You are on a journey that holds the promise of ever-increasing freedom from unconsciously held patterns residual from childhood. You can finally acknowledge with affection the good boy or girl you thought you'd left in the past.

The next time you scan the environment comparing yourself to others, take in hand the one who is trying so hard to please others. Then tell the anxious child who still lives inside of you that it's finally time for recess.

OCTOBER

First Week of October

The secret is to be able to want one thing, to seek one thing, to organize the resources of one's life around a single end; and slowly, surely, the life becomes one with that end.

HOWARD THURMAN

You have a vision for how life could be for you, and through all the obstacles, disappointments, and naysayers you have persevered. It took more than you knew you had in you because genuine spiritual and psychological growth often turns out to be a last resort. We do everything we can for as long as possible to protect our illusion of control until every denial, bypass, and shortcut around facing reality has come to a dead end.

In breaking old dependencies, your old coping strategies must be definitively defeated by bad news, crises, and circumstances that don't meet your expectations. Your nerves get shot first, then you ride through waves of panic, and finally you wash up on a distant shore, tongue out and panting. There is, at last, a heartrending arrival to acceptance. What joy when you come to realize it is all in service of something, and that in the end it has proven to be worth the struggle.

In retrospect you can see clearly that there has been a trajectory to your life—an organizing principle around which genuine growth transpired. This forward movement did not come about without sacrifice. By being willing to do whatever it would take, you discovered you are stronger than you thought. Now on the far side of midlife you have access to previously untapped wells of freedom, love, and courage.

So here's a salute to everything you have endured, everything you've released, and everything you have become. Yes, it's taken longer than you would have hoped, but as it turns out, you are right on time.

Second Week of October

As you review the recent past and the week ahead, do you view yourself as someone who is inspired yet relaxed going through your days? Or are you driven, worn out by your commitments? This week is a good time to take an inventory of the pace of your life and what it is you are working so hard to achieve. An apocryphal tale provides guidance.

One day Alexander the Great was leading his troops through India when he spotted a saint sitting serenely on the banks of the river.

"I wish I could be sitting there as you are, enjoying the sun," Alexander said.

"Where are you going?" the saint replied.

"I'm going to fight one more battle and then I will return to sit beside you."

The saint looked deeply into Alexander's eyes and said, "If what you really want in the end is to sit here with me enjoying the river, why don't you just do it now?"

As the story teaches, an inspired life has nothing to do with how much or how little you choose to take on. It doesn't matter what others think, or whether or not you believe you're fulfilling what you thought was your potential.

You say you want serenity? To savor the moment? To have more time to meditate and self-nurture? If that's what you really want in the end, why not do it now?

Third Week of October

Positive change rarely feels natural or right at first. Growth summons you to ride out the discomfort anyway. Ramifications and aftershocks are not proof that you've failed. They are proof that there are people in your life who preferred you powerless and unhappy.

The people who got used to your being one way will not necessarily like the new you who is learning to set boundaries, demand respect, and be heard. If you allow them to cast guilt or doubt, you can easily find yourself questioning whether you're just making trouble and reminiscing about how good things used to be (but in truth, rarely were). If you find yourself wishing you could make things go back to the way they were, you are undoubtedly denying how much of that peace was bought at the cost of walking on eggshells.

Here's a formula that will empower your feet to keep moving forward as you journey through the rockier stretches of individuation: First, honor yourself for taking on this self-appraisal. Acknowledge any guilt or shame you are carrying on behalf of others, then subtract from this the truth, which is either that you are already good enough and/or that your imperfect humanity is forgivable. Also subtract the sobering fact that not everybody has your best interests at heart, possibly including a few of those for whom you care deeply.

Your summation can be measured in percentages, weights, or quantities. However you work the numbers, the answer will always be the same: infinite, for this is the value of your self-worth.

Fourth Week of October

There are mornings when the sun rises, just as surely as every day of your life, but behind a thick veil of clouds. You have tossed and turned your concerns over all night long to no avail, and now you must make a decision. Do you dig deep to find it within you to push through anyway and get on with your day, or do you submit to the moment that is too big for you to control?

If the answer comes, do it. There is no right or wrong. Some days you may throw on your protective gear and venture forth bravely to do what is yours to do. Other days you can do nothing more than make it to your favorite chair and curl up under your comforter.

But there is a third option—you can ask for help. There is no shame to admitting you can't do this on your own. If no one comes to mind, you can pray to the Divine. "Help me to remember that you are with me always, even when I feel most alone and needy. And even if my faith in myself has faltered, I trust that you've got this."

Exactly when you feel the least able and willing is the most potent moment for prayer. Whether you believe your words will be heard or not, even acting "as if" is the initiation of a turning point. Trust this much, and when the first ray of light peeks through you will remember that help is already on the way.

Fifth Week of October
or Bonus Reading

*Even with the highest development
and liberation, the person comes up
against the real despair of the human
condition. Indeed, because of that
development his eyes are opened to the
reality of things; there is no turning
back to the comforts of a secure and
armored life.*

ERNEST BECKER

You have always pictured yourself to be a seeker of meaning. This quest has defined your journey in search of a singular truth that would help you make sense of things. But you have also thought of yourself as a truth-teller, and the older you become, the more reality grows to be nearly more than you can bear. At times this feels like regression, leaving you to ponder whether things have really become that much worse—politics, the environment, human nature—or is it that you have become less able to take refuge in illusion?

What is spiritual aging if not about becoming increasingly willing to be honest with yourself about what you had previously denied? Inconveniently awake, one can no longer find the gift or lesson, let alone the meaning of life, in environmental disaster, endless wars, humanitarian crises, anything about many politicians, and really, virtually all the news. Rather than grow despondent or check out altogether, your only recourse is to ask the philosopher's perennial question: *How, then, are we to live?*

Ernest Becker, in his 1973 classic *Denial of Death,* offers insight that provides a path through the wilderness. Becker's counsel is to face the truth leaving nothing out, then mitigate your despair with something you can control. In other words, a project. Becker notes that by doing so, one's life becomes "a duty of cosmic heroism." Easier said than done, to be both a seeker of meaning and a truth-teller is not for the weakhearted.

How to make a start? Begin anywhere with anything. Is there something that interests you that you'd judged too insignificant or too difficult? Stop worrying about whether it's really your true purpose, or whether it's enough. Choose something and dig in with an open mind and heart. Prepare to be surprised as you discover that in doing so, you set forces in motion that will bring you fresh hope, insights, and courage. Hold the reins of your project loose and let it flow. Create your own meaning, one word, one stitch, one interesting thing at a time.

NOVEMBER

First Week of November

You have learned life's lessons about surrender and acceptance, some perhaps a little too well. Because you are committed to aging consciously, your ego has learned how to take life as it comes.

But have you forgotten that it's also okay to hope? When was the last time you asked yourself, *What is my heart's desire?* How often do you give yourself permission to ask for what it is you really want? A story adapted from William James teaches us about hope.

Two mountaineers are nearing the peak of the mountain and there is no turning back, but ahead lies a dangerous chasm. The only way forward is a terrifying leap. The first climber is frozen in fear, sure he's doomed. The second knows it will be a stretch but believes that at the very least, intention, hope, and faith will put him in a more optimal frame of mind to make it across than would terror and mistrust.

drives you. You, old friend, are one of the few in our ambition-driven society to have broken free. Yes, it is you, dear one, who has ascended to the peak of adult and spiritual development. But still it is incumbent upon you to remind even your most humbled self not to take your nobodyness too seriously. A story adapted from Geri Larkin goes like this.

After chanting Buddha's name for years, an old woman suddenly sees behind the veil of all of life's illusions, the light of truth flooding over her. She can't wait to share the news of her awakening with her Zen Master Hakuin. Arriving to his side she tells him that her whole body is shining with great enlightenment.

"Oh really?" he says. "And is this great light also shining up your butt?"

Even though the old woman is tiny, she pushes him over, shouting:

"Well I can see you still have work to do yourself, old man!"

Which one do you think will have the better chance of surviving? No matter how much you may want something, there are no guarantees. But the author notes, "To believe is greatly to your advantage."

Second Week of November

How far you've come from the days you needed fancy titles, prestige, and accomplishments to prove to the world that you are a somebody!

This week, recall earlier in life just how long you had to struggle to build an identity you hoped would provide you safe passage. Inventory all your attempts to secure status for yourself through the decades leading up to the recent past. Keep in mind we're talking less about what you set as your goal—be it having a bestseller, moving to the best neighborhood, or whatever you deemed essential to becoming somebody— but your motivation. It's one thing to do something because you find it fulfilling. It's another thing to go against the grain of what your heart is telling you because you're still seeking others' approval in an attempt to ratify your identity.

You did, indeed, become somebody—at least for awhile. But it isn't long before no matter how much effort you bring to the table, your identities begin slipping away. "Formerly," "Emeritus," "Retired" find their ways onto your resume. Your grandchild, who imbued your life with meaning by going to Harvard, drops out to surf. Your book goes out of print. And even if you could continue riding your ego bareback through life, sustaining being a somebody at the cost of your own authenticity eventually grows tired.

Here in the Land of Old Souls, having left so much of your old identity behind, you have discovered that there is something much better than being a somebody. It's called freedom, and comes only to those of us who are aging consciously. Released from the yoke of how others define you, you can be at once anything, everything, and nothing.

Now that you realize you don't need to do or be anything in particular to be beloved and how little it really takes for you to feel safe and content, the fear of being a nobody no longer

The two burst out laughing and are so over-taken by joy "that they dance and dance and dance—awakeness meeting awakeness."

Yes, this is a good week to celebrate how far you've come. But this is even a better week to have a good laugh about it, because nobody understands the irony of the achievement of humility better than you.

Third Week of November

Some days things go awry and nobody is more surprised than you when not only do you feel bad, but you top it off by turning on yourself for not feeling better. You believe you should be able to bypass the negativity by rising above it or letting it go. Ironically, the higher your spiritual aspirations, the greater your tendency to judge negative feelings as beneath you.

When you get triggered by emotions you thought you'd processed years ago, it feels like self-betrayal. You get lost in them as they pile up on one another. But what if you tendered just enough belief in yourself to view even your rawest emotions as the call for discernment, not judgment?

You're sad. But is this really a case of self-pity you know better than to indulge, or authentic grief that needs only to be endured?

You're angry. Is this the petulance of a child

who needs to be taken in hand, or the legitimate summons to respond to an injustice or deceit?

You're hurt. Are you allowing fear not facts to provide the interpretation of events, or has the time come to set healthy boundaries?

Instead of flapping broken wings in the fruitless effort to rise above bad feelings, what if you tendered yourself the courtesy of asking whether this is really a matter of the descent you fear or of growth?

It is the most authentic expression of your spirituality that will answer the question honestly. And in the end, it will not be your feelings, whether bad or good, but grace that will show the way through.

Fourth Week of November

The search for meaning drove you for decades. You thought of life as a puzzle to be solved and the prize would be the discovery of your higher purpose.

When you were young it was others who attempted to answer the question of meaning for you. Following their lead, you may have been expected to go into the family business, cure cancer, run for office, win an Academy Award, or become a priest.

Some of us realized early on that others' desire to determine our life's purpose was not a good fit. We were the ones who were labeled rebels or failures. "You'll never amount to anything" was the refrain that accompanied our coming of age. Others of us complied and found ourselves praised and respected, while feeling hollow and unsatisfied.

Meanwhile, life goes on. You got educated,

got your first job. You made choices about getting married, having children. You decided where you would live, which hobbies, activities, and causes you would adopt. Some of your decisions worked out fine, others not so much. But still, you persevered.

All the while you were building memories: a lifetime full of simple joys and unavoidable losses. There was celebration, crisis, joy, sadness, every possible emotion, but through it all something miraculous transpired: You fell in love with your life.

Now that you are old you have finally come to realize that there's a better question to ask yourself than what is the purpose of life. It is simply this: *What would I like to do today?*

Fifth Week of November
or Bonus Reading

If you obey all the rules,
you miss all the fun.

KATHARINE HEPBURN

One of the gifts of spiritual aging is that you finally realize you have the power to stop wasting valuable energy either seeking approval or proving how much better you are than others. In this new stage of psychological and spiritual maturity you are finally free to reclaim your innate capacity to experience, express, and act on authentic feelings.

Drawing upon a new level of emotional maturity, you have learned when it's worth speaking your mind and when it is more prudent or gracious to keep it to yourself. You are less manipulable, more forgiving, slower to judge, and more compassionate with your own as well as other's foibles and shortcomings. You are increasingly less prone to knee-jerk reactivity to the past, as well as fears about the future. This is the essence of true freedom. And this is just the start.

There are a lot of us waking up to this new level of freedom simultaneously. At last we are spending less time walking on eggshells, feeling unwarranted shame or embarrassment, providing long explanations, and playing defense. In its place all that's left on your to-do list is one thing: relish the moment you realize you're done apologizing.

DECEMBER

First Week of December

This week, pause to acknowledge the unpalatable truth that the well-worn persona you cultivated over the many decades is no longer functioning as you once hoped it would, no longer offering the cover of protection as part of an ongoing, diligent work in progress. But this week your response to self-exposure can be different, a leaning into the changes rather than defending against them.

It's true that you don't know what the future holds for you, but this is no different from before, when you'd expended tremendous effort trying to wrestle the challenges associated with aging into something manageable. How much energy have you wasted looking for a way to protect yourself?

Let go of the illusion of your control, and the only thing you sacrifice is the exhaustion of wasted effort and disappointment with your outcomes. In their place you can let yourself flow into whatever life is to be for you, moment by moment. Do this and life becomes an adventure with surprising twists and turns.

In his novel *Exit Ghost*, Philip Roth presents us with a character who got the message.

"I was learning at seventy-one what it is to be deranged. Proving that self-discovery wasn't over after all. Proving that the drama that is associated usually with the young as they fully begin to enter life . . . can also startle and lay siege to the aged."

At times life is cruel, other times magnificent. But regardless, you no longer need to steel yourself against the future because in loosening your grip you will receive the answer to the only essential concern: the question of your lovability. Once you experience the unconditional love that is the byproduct of acceptance, saving yourself is no longer necessary.

This week allow yourself to go all in on who

you really are, conditions and all. Avail yourself anew to self-exposure by saying these simple but powerful words: *I am not being careful anymore. I am being myself.*

So here, at last, is the way forward you've been seeking, for now you are no longer growing old. You are growing free.

Second Week of December

You have worked hard and long to make an arrival, and here at last you are. Admittedly, this is not the grand transcendence you imagined but rather a soft landing into something far more grounded— the joy of simple comfort. Your favorite chair, for instance. Perhaps you are curled up in it now. Your special candle, the scent that caresses your soul. The room temperature is just right. There is no place else you have to be, nowhere to go, nothing more to achieve.

Comfort, itself, is your destination and your reward for all the fortitude it took you to shed all that had separated you from the simple sweetness of divine love. Those were the still hours before dawn when you gradually traded confessing your shortcomings to tell the whole truth about yourself—the good things, too.

Comfort is a culmination, the simple choices you make to avail yourself of days and nights illuminated by the natural light of your deepest being, a reflection of God's love. Your pillow. A hand-knit throw. There is comfort in surrendering to the truth of your beauty, all that had been behind the mask now revealed and embraced.

Comfort is your celebration. When you touch such moments, all the rest—the missteps, transgressions, failings—are no longer front and center. Rather, they take their place at your side as you come to cherish the whole of your life, delighted with your part in it.

In love, the work is complete and comfort is your home.

Third Week of December

After waiting for what seemed an eternity, the old man reached the head of the line where he cowered before an enormous gate. His eyes were so full of tears he could not read the sign. Screwing up the courage to speak, he asked the gatekeeper:

"Where am I? I know I died. But is this the gate to heaven or to hell?"

The gatekeeper replied, "Tell me first, where are those tears coming from?"

The old man stopped to think and a stream of memories flooded over him. Immediately, he thought of the old woman left behind, the many decades they had walked through life together, hand in hand. He thought of the joys and hardships, so much that they had faced together and overcome. He thought of his friends and family, favorite pets and places. He had experienced crises and he had experienced joy and every possible emotion.

There were those times he'd lost his temper or did something he later regretted, and even more times he'd apologized. He had not always succeeded at everything he attempted and surely there was so much more he'd hoped to accomplish. But now all he felt was sorrow for all he had lost.

The gatekeeper witnessed it all and when the old man finally paused, he told him, "Only one who has loved so greatly can feel so much pain. Before I answer your question as to whether you are standing before the gate to heaven or to hell, you must answer one for me. Have you been blessed or have you been cursed?"

So startled was he by the gatekeeper's words, the old man's eyes suddenly cleared and he had his answer.

"If it were a curse," he declared, "I would give none of it back."

With that his fear departed, leaving behind only the bittersweet love in his heart. Had he always intended to give life his best? And was he not already blessed? He no longer needed to be able to read the word above the gate to know his destiny. At that moment the gatekeeper threw open the doors and waved him through.

Fourth Week of December

You are quickly approaching the end of another year of diligent inner work, and you are on the cusp of the initiation of a new stage of growth. It hasn't always been easy but you persevered. You have learned that your ability to progress is not dependent upon your objective circumstances, but rather the profound shift in your perspective that your diligent internal work made possible.

You answered the call to do whatever it would take to increase your consciousness, leaving nothing out. This included making peace with your past, rectifying everything within your power, and tendering unconditional love for the whole of your life, even that which you do not remember with pleasure. Apparently wasted time, foolish mistakes, misplaced priorities, and nearly every size, manner, and shape of regret . . . how wondrous to be reviewing your history from the elevated vantage point of forgiveness, acceptance, and gratitude.

You have come to appreciate that there is efficiency to the practice of spiritual aging, in which everything that took place throughout the arc of your life can be understood to have happened for a purpose. By healing your relationship with yourself you have come to realize that you've never been particularly bad and that you no longer have to run and rerun the story of your victimhood. You no longer need to feed the lie of unworthiness that once fueled your ambition and your envy, nor look outside yourself for protection from life.

You are privileged to have lived long enough to witness your own legacy: the long-sought experience of unconditional love. In this place of culmination you are quietly harvesting your heart's desire, celebrating the goodness you have always wanted to experience for yourself and sharing it with those for whom you care.

You're beloved. You're authentic. You're enough. The time has come to unfurl the wings of your spirit and soar.

Fifth Week of December
or Bonus Reading

As you approach the transition to a new year, celebrate all the joy you've derived from the expansion of your consciousness these past fifty-two weeks. Here are but a few of the many things you now know about yourself and life:

1. When you review the past it isn't denial to cherry pick the beautiful moments—and there were many!
2. Seeking the acceptance of an unhealthy tribe hurts everyone. You can relate to the tribe without becoming immersed in it.
3. By standing firm, your authentic self serves as a doorway to freedom for others to become more fully themselves, as well.
4. The voice that says you are unworthy of fulfilling your heart's desire is always unreliable.

5. You are a beautiful soul who is not afraid to love deeply. Even if you emerged from toxic programming, you aspired to giving and receiving love unconditionally, and you succeeded.

6. You may not be able to be near those you love all the time, but you can love them all the time.

7. Being fun, flowing, appreciative, simple is a choice you make every time you listen to the loving voice in your heart instead of the critic.

8. You are not how you look but what you see, and what you see is love and beauty.

9. You can be kind and it is your pleasure to share from your essential abundance.

10. Life is an ongoing journey but when every step is taken in the present moment, it is also an arrival.

There is so much about you and your life worth celebrating and you are justified in counting on continued growth toward wholeness through the year to come. However, the mystics advise us not to concern ourselves with how to live from this new place but to simply be present to the larger truth one week, one day, one moment at a time, trusting that all else are details that will work themselves out.

There is nothing more than this you need to do. And in this spirit of faith and love, we close this year not with answers but a question: What if you were to live your aging as a fearless experiment, with purpose enough to just do one thing that interests you after another?

This is your final reading of the year. You've accomplished much but there is always more life to be lived and lessons to be learned, so see you again next week as we turn not only once again but ever more deeply to the beginning of a new year.

Well Done, Old Friend

Week by week, you've come to the end of a calendar year devoted to spiritual aging!

What's next?

Turn back to the very first reading and start over again with a fresh perspective in your new circumstances. Because, old soul, by now you know that as much as you have accomplished, there's always something more.

To deepen your experience, consider starting a Spiritual Aging Study and Support Group (SASS) with friends to discuss the readings. You are also invited to join my online inner circle of old souls, engaging with me and like-minded members on an ongoing basis. (For details, see "How to Stay Connected" on page 343.)

Or, on the other hand, do whatever you'd

like because you know what? You deserve it.

Here's to living every day in wonder, joy, and mystery.

And as the mystics like to say: You've got this!

How to Stay Connected

Let's stay connected at my website
CarolOrsborn.com
There you will find links to free content, including a self-guided retreat, access to the *Fierce with Age* archives, and a calendar of events under the tab "Offerings."

To receive *The Spiritual Aging Study Guide* week-by-week in your inbox, you are invited to join my online Spiritual Aging Study and Support Group (SASS) at SpiritualAging.substack.com. As a member, you will have the opportunity to engage online with me and fellow members on an ongoing basis.

More Ways to Connect

Email: carol@carolorsborn.com
Facebook: Facebook.com/FierceWithAge
YouTube: @CarolOrsborn6775

Sources of Inspiration
and Quotes

Achenbaum, W. Andrew. *Crossing Frontiers: Gerontology Emerges as a Science.* New York: Cambridge University Press, 1995.

Anonymous. *One Day at a Time in Al-Anon.* Virginia Beach, VA: Al-Anon Family Group Headquarters, 2000.

Anthony, Bolton. *Second Journeys: The Dance of Spirit in Later Life.* Chapel Hill, NC: Second Journeys Publications, 2013.

Atchley, Robert C. *Spirituality and Aging.* Baltimore, MD: Johns Hopkins University Press, 2009.

Bierman, Harold, and Donald Schnedeker. *Insights for Managers from Confucius to Gandhi.* New York: Modern Library, 1938.

Blondin, Sarah. *Heart Minded: How to Hold Yourself and Others in Love.* Boulder, CO: Sounds True, 2020.

Broyard, Anatole. *Intoxicated by My Illness: And Other Writings on Life and Death*. New York: Fawcett, Columbine. 1992.

Campbell, Joseph. *The Hero with a Thousand Faces*. San Rafael, CA: New World Library, 2008.

Campbell, Joseph, and Michael Toms. *An Open Life: Joseph Campbell in Conversation with Michael Toms*. New York: Harper Perennial, 1990.

Chittister, Joan. *The Gift of Years: Growing Older Gracefully*. New York: BlueBridge, 2008.

Chodron, Pema, *Start Where You Are: A Guide to Compassionate Living*. Boston: Shambhala Publishing, 1994.

Cobb, John B., Jr., and David Ray Griffin. *Process Theology: An Introductory Exposition*. Philadelphia: Westminster Press, 1976.

Ellis, Havelock. *Studies in the Psychology of Sex, Volume 1*. New York: Random House, 1942.

Erikson, Erik H. *The Life Cycle Completed: A Review*. New York: W. W. Norton & Company, 1982.

Fowler, J. W. *Stages of Faith: The Psychology of Human Development and the Quest for Meaning*. New York: Harper & Row, 1981.

Frankl, Viktor. *Man's Search for Meaning*. Boston: Beacon Press, 1962.

Freed, Jann E. *Breadcrumb Legacy: How Great Leaders Live a Life Worth Remembering*. New York: Routledge, 2023.

Goldman, Connie. *Who Am I: Now That I'm Not Who I Was: Conversations with Women in Mid-Life and the Years Beyond*. Minneapolis: Nodin, 2009.

———. *Wisdom from Those in Care: Conversations, Insights, and Inspiration*. Minneapolis: Partners in Caregiving Project, 2018.

Green, Brent, with Carol Orsborn, David Cogswell, Richard Adler, Bob Moses, Jed Diamond, Greg Dobbs, and Robert William Case. *1969: Are You Still Listening?* Denver, CO: Brent Green & Assoc., 2019.

Gunn, Robert Jingen. *Journey into Emptiness: Dogen, Merton, Jung, and the Quest for Transformation*. Mahwah, NJ: Paulist Press, 2000.

Hillman, James. *The Force of Character and the Lasting Life*. New York: Random House, 1999.

Hoblitzelle, Olivia Ames. *Aging with Wisdom: Reflections, Stories, & Teachings*. Rhinebeck, NY: Monkfish Publishing, 2017.

Hollis, James. *Finding Meaning in the Second Half of Life: How to Finally, Really Grow Up.* New York: Gotham Books, 2005.

———. *Living between Worlds: Finding Personal Resilience in Changing Times.* Boulder, CO: Sounds True, 2020.

———. *Swamplands of the Soul: New Life in Dismal Places.* Scarborough, Ontario: Inner City Books, 1996.

Huxley, Aldous. *The Doors of Perception: Includes Heaven and Hell.* New York: Harper, 1954.

James, William. *The Varieties of Religious Experience: A Study in Human Nature.* New York: Collier, 1961.

Jeffers, Susan. *Feel the Fear . . . and Do It Anyway.* 20th Anniversary edition. New York: Ballantine Books, 2006.

Jung, C. G. *Memories, Dreams, Reflections.* New York: Vintage Books, 1989.

Lamott, Anne. *Almost Everything: Notes on Hope.* New York: Riverhead Books, 2018.

Lew, Alan. *This Is Real and You Are Completely Unprepared: The Days of Awe as a Journey of Transformation.* Boston: Little, Brown, 2003.

Lustbader, Wendy. *Life Gets Better: The Unexpected Pleasures of Growing Older.* New York: Jeremy P. Tarcher/Penguin, 2011.

Kapur, Kamla K., *The Privilege of Aging: Savoring the Fullness of Life.* Rochester, VT: Park Street Press, 2024.

Kroeber, Theodora. *Ishi in Two Worlds: A Biography of the Last Wild Indian in North America.* Berkeley: University of California Press, 2011.

Kuner, Susan, Carol Orsborn, Linda Quigley, and Karen Stroup. *Speak the Language of Healing: Living with Breast Cancer without Going to War.* Foreword by Jean Shinoda Bolen, M.D. Berkeley, CA: Conari Press, 1997.

Laarman, Peter. "Among School Children." *Reflections: Test of Time/The Art of Aging.* New Haven, CT: Yale Divinity School, 2013.

Larkin, Geri. "Close to the Ground: The Secret of Abiding Joy." *Spirituality + Health* (Nov./Dec. 2015) and online.

Lin Yutang. *The Wisdom of Confucius.* New York: Random House, 1938

Merton, Thomas. *Echoing Silence: Thomas Merton on the Vocation of Writing.* New York: New Seeds, 2008.

———. *No Man Is an Island*. New York: Image/ Doubleday, 1955.

———. *The Seven Storey Mountain: An Autobiography of Faith*. New York: Harcourt, 1948.

———. *The Silent Life*. New York: Dell, 1957.

Metzger, Bruce M., and Roland E. Murphy, eds. *The New Oxford Annotated Bible*. New York: Oxford University Press, 1991.

Moody, Harry R., and David Carroll. *The Five Stages of the Soul: Charting the Spiritual Passages That Shape Our Lives*. New York: Anchor Books, 1997.

Niebuhr, Reinhold. Quoted in *AA Grapevine: The International Journal of Alcoholics Anonymous* (January 1950): 6–7.

Nouwen, Henri J. M., and Walter J. Gaffney. *Aging: The Fulfillment of Life*. New York: Image Books, 1976.

O'Donohue, John. *To Bless the Space between Us: A Book of Blessings*. New York: Crown Publishing, 2008.

Orsborn, Carol. *Angelica's Last Breath*. Nashville, TN: Fierce with Age Press, 2018.

———. *The Art of Resilience: 100 Paths to Wisdom and Strength in an Uncertain World*. New York: Three Rivers Press (Random House), 1997.

———. *Fierce with Age: Chasing God and Squirrels in Brooklyn*. Nashville, TN: Turner Publishing, 2013.

———. *How Would Confucius Ask for a Raise: One Hundred Enlightened Solutions for Tough Business Problems*. New York: Avon, 1994.

———. *The Making of an Old Soul: Aging as the Fulfillment of Life's Promise*. Amherst, MA: White River Press, 2021.

———. *Nothing Left Unsaid: Words to Help You and Your Loved Ones through the Hardest Time*. Berkeley, CA: Conari Press, 2001.

———. *Older, Wiser, Fiercer: The Wisdom Collection*. Nashville, TN: Fierce with Age Press, 2020.

———. *Solved by Sunset: The Self-Guided Intuitive Decision-Making Retreat*. New York: Harmony, 1996.

Otto, Rudolf. *The Idea of the Holy: An Inquiry into the Non-rational Factor in the Idea of the Divine and Its Relation to the Rational*. London: Oxford University Press, 1958.

Palmer, Parker J. *On the Brink of Everything: Grace, Gravity & Getting Old*. Oakland, CA: Berrett-Koehler Publishers, 2018.

Pevny, Ron. *Conscious Living, Conscious Aging: Embrace and Savor Your Next Chapter*. New York: Atria Books/Beyond Words, 2014.

Ram Dass. *Still Here: Embracing Aging, Changing, and Dying*. New York: Penguin Books, 2000.

Rhiannon, Felice. *A Vibrant Life: Yoga in the Middle Years and Beyond*. Victoria, Canada: Trafford Publishing, 2008.

Robinson, John C. *The Three Secrets of Aging: A Radical Guide*. Winchester, UK: O-Books, 2012.

Rohr, Richard. *Falling Upward: A Spirituality for the Two Halves of Life*. San Francisco: Jossey-Bass, 2011.

Roof, Wade Clark. *A Generation of Seekers: The Spiritual Journeys of the Baby Boom Generation*. San Francisco: HarperSanFrancisco, 1994.

Sarton, May. *At Eighty-Two: A Journal.* New York: Norton, 1996.

———. *Journal of a Solitude.* New York: Norton, 1992.

Schachter-Shalomi, Zalman. *From Age-ing to Sage-ing: A Revolutionary Approach to Growing Older.* New York: Oxford University Press, 1997.

Scott-Maxwell, Florida. *The Measure of My Days: One Woman's Vivid, Enduring Celebration of Life and Aging.* New York: Penguin Books, 1968.

Shapiro, Rami. *Recovery—The Sacred Art: The Twelve Steps as Spiritual Practice*. Nashville, TN: SkyLight Paths Publishing, 2009.

Sheehy, Gail. *New Passages: Mapping Your Life Across Time*. New York: Random House, 1995.

Singer, Isaac Bashevis. *The Family Moskat*. New York: Farrar, Straus, and Giroux, 2007.

Singer, Michael. *The Untethered Soul: The Journey Beyond Yourself*. Oakland, CA: New Harbinger, 2007.

Singh, Kathleen Dowling. *The Grace in Aging: Awaken as You Grow Older*. Somerville, MA: Wisdom Publications, 2014.

Storr, Anthony. *Solitude: A Return to the Self*. New York: Free Press, 1988.

Thibault, Jane Marie, and Richard L. Morgan. *Pilgrimage into the Last Third of Life: 7 Gateways to Spiritual Growth*. Nashville, TN: Upper Room Books, 2012.

Thurman, Howard. *Disciplines of the Spirit*. Richmond, IN: Friends United Press, 1963.

Tolstoy, Leo. *Childhood, Boyhood, Youth*. New York: Penguin Classics, 2012.

———. *The Death of Ivan Ilyich*. New York: Bantam Classic, 2004

Traherne, Thomas. *Centuries of Meditations*. Grand Rapids, MI: Christian Classics Ethereal Library, 1908.

Underhill, Evelyn. *The Mystic Way: The Role of Mysticism in the Christian Life*. London: Forgotten Books, 2013.

Weber, Robert L., and Carol Orsborn. *The Spirituality of Age: A Seeker's Guide to Growing Older*. Rochester, VT: Inner Traditions, 2015.

Wieseltier, Leon. *Kaddish*. New York: Alfred A. Knopf, 1998.

Whitman, Walt. *Specimen Days and Collect*. Philadelphia: David McKay, 1882–83.

Wilhelm, Richard, trans., and Cary F. Baynes, trans. *The I Ching: Or Book of Changes*. Princeton, NJ: Princeton University Press, 1967.

Yalom, Irvin D. *Staring at the Sun: Overcoming the Dread of Death*. San Francisco: Jossey-Bass, 2008.

Yudron, Gaea. "Full Moon, Summer Solstice: Contemplating the Archetypes." *Sage's Play* (June 20, 2016).

Zweig, Connie. *The Inner Work of Age: Shifting from Role to Soul*. Rochester, VT: Inner Traditions, 2022.

About the Author

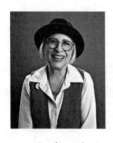

Carol Orsborn, Ph.D., is a recognized thought leader in the field of spiritual aging. She has written more than 35 books and her work has been translated into 18 languages.

Orsborn's two most recent books are *The Making of an Old Soul: Aging as the Fulfillment of Life's Promise* (White River Press, 2021) and *Older, Wiser, Fiercer* (Fierce with Age Press, 2020), which has been on bestseller lists in the aging category consistently since its publication. Her groundbreaking book *The Spirituality of Age: A Seeker's Guide to Growing Older* (Inner Traditions, 2015), coauthored with Harvard psychologist Robert Weber, Ph.D., won Gold in the Nautilus Book

Awards in the category of Aging Consciously. She has also been a finalist in the Jewish Book Awards.

Orsborn leads an interactive online membership community study and support group centered on her book *Spiritual Aging: Weekly Reflections for Embracing Life* at SpiritualAging.substack.com, blogs regularly at CarolOrsborn.com, and is chief archivist of *Fierce with Age: The Digest of Boomer Wisdom, Inspiration and Spirituality*, housed at her website. She leads a global online study and support group based on *Spiritual Aging* for Sageing International, the leading organization in the field of conscious aging. She also leads groups and retreats for women studying her latest work for Spirit of Sophia, an in-person and online women's spirituality center.

For the past forty years Orsborn has been a compelling voice of her generation, interviewed on *Oprah, The Today Show,* and *CBS Morning News* and in *The New York Times, Washington Post,* and *The Wall Street Journal.* She speaks regularly to association and industry groups on the Boomer generation. Past engagements include the American Society of Aging, What's Next Boomer Summit, Omega Institute, Vanderbilt University Medical Center, the Positive Aging Conference, and The Shift Network. Orsborn's original work on resilience, based on her Random House book, *The Art of Resilience*, has been presented to such corporate clients as the Walt Disney Company, ABC Broadcast Network, Southern California Edison, and Wellpoint.

In the late 1980s Orsborn founded Super-women's Anonymous. News of her organization, followed by her first book, *Enough Is Enough: Exploding the Myth of Having It All* (Putnam), was credited as a progenitor of both the simplic-ity and work/life balance movements. Thirty-five books followed chronicling the challenges her generation has faced and the stereotypes they've defied as they've transited from early parent-hood through midlife crisis and onto the largely unexplored terrain of conscious aging. Her books have won praise from a wide range of authors, critics, and experts, including Gail Sheehy, Peter Senge, Harold Kushner, and Gerald Jampolski.

A Phi Beta Kappa graduate of UC Berkeley, Orsborn received her master of theological studies from Vanderbilt Divinity School and a doctorate in history and critical theory of religion from the Graduate School of Religion, Vanderbilt University. Her area of specialization is adult and spiritual development and life stage theory. She has done postgraduate work in spiritual guidance at the New Seminary of Interfaith Studies in Manhattan and the Los Angeles Spirituality Center at Mount St. Mary's University. She has served on the faculties of Georgetown University, Vanderbilt University's Leadership Development Center, Loyola Marymount University, and the Doctoral Program in Organizational Leadership at Pepperdine University as well as on the Board of Visitors of Vanderbilt Divinity School.

Orsborn lives in Nashville, Tennessee, and Toronto, Canada, with her husband of fifty-five years, Dan Orsborn, and their dog, Winnie. She has an extended family including her two beloved grown children, their spouses, and two grandsons.

Subject Index

Welcome to the *Spiritual Aging* subject index. Scan the alphabetical list below to be directed to select reflections addressing whatever mood, issue, or interest is calling to you now.